The A to Z of Pregnancy & Child Birth

Samantha Taylor

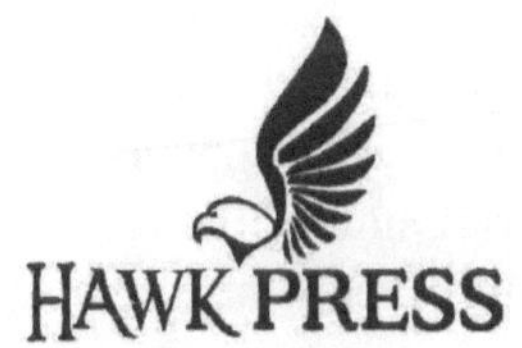

HAWK PRESS

Published by

Hawk Press
4836/24, Ansari Road, Daryaganj
New Delhi – 110 002
Phones : 9643330713, 91-11-23278618, 91-11-35676207
E-mail: thehawkpress@gmail.com
www.thehawkpress.com

Contents

Preface

Pregnancy, also known as gestation, is the time during which one or more offspring develops inside a woman. A multiple pregnancy involves more than one offspring, such as with twins. Pregnancy usually occurs by sexual intercourse, but can also occur through assisted reproductive technology procedures. A pregnancy may end in a live birth, a spontaneous miscarriage, an induced abortion, or a stillbirth. Childbirth typically occurs around 40 weeks from the start of the last menstrual period (LMP).

Pregnancy, process and series of changes that take place in a woman's organs and tissues as a result of a developing fetus. The entire process from fertilization to birth takes an average of 266–270 days, or about nine months.

Pregnancy occurs when a sperm fertilizes an egg after it's released from the ovary during ovulation. The fertilized egg then travels down into the uterus, where implantation occurs. A successful implantation results in pregnancy.

On average, a full-term pregnancy lasts 40 weeks. There are many factors that can affect a pregnancy. Women who receive an early pregnancy diagnosis and prenatal care are more likely to experience a healthy pregnancy and give birth to a healthy baby.

Knowing what to expect during the full pregnancy term is important for monitoring both your health and the health of the baby. If you'd like to prevent pregnancy, there are also effective forms of birth control you should keep in mind.

A new individual is created when the elements of a potent sperm merge with those of a fertile ovum, or egg. Before this union both the spermatozoon (sperm) and the ovum have migrated for considerable distances in order to achieve their union. A number of actively motile spermatozoa are deposited in the vagina, pass through the uterus, and invade the uterine (fallopian) tube, where they surround the ovum. The ovum has arrived there after extrusion from its follicle, or capsule, in the ovary. After it enters the tube, the ovum loses its outer layer of cells as a result of action by substances in the spermatozoa and from the lining of the tubal wall. Loss of the outer layer of the ovum allows a number of spermatozoa to penetrate the egg's surface. Only one spermatozoon, however, normally becomes the fertilizing organism. Once it has entered the substance of the ovum, the nuclear head of this spermatozoon separates from its tail. The tail gradually disappears, but the head with its nucleus survives. As it travels toward the nucleus of the ovum (at this stage called the female pronucleus), the head enlarges and becomes the male pronucleus. The two pronuclei meet in the centre of the ovum, where their threadlike chromatin material organizes into chromosomes.

This book provides not only the information of how to have a baby but also tells how to maintain your body through exercise, learn relaxing and breathing techniques, adopt labour positions to facilitate childbirth and take care of him or her.

—Editor

1

Introduction

Pregnancy, also known as gestation, is the time during which one or more offspring develops inside a woman. A multiple pregnancy involves more than one offspring, such as with twins. Pregnancy usually occurs by sexual intercourse, but can also occur through assisted reproductive technology procedures. A pregnancy may end in a live birth, a spontaneous miscarriage, an induced abortion, or a stillbirth. Childbirth typically occurs around 40 weeks from the start of the last menstrual period (LMP). This is just over nine months (gestational age)—where each month averages 31 days. When using fertilization age it is about 38 weeks. An embryo is the developing offspring during the first eight weeks following fertilization, (ten weeks' gestational age) after which, the term *fetus* is used until birth. Signs and symptoms of early pregnancy may include missed periods, tender breasts, morning sickness (nausea and vomiting), hunger, and frequent urination. Pregnancy may be confirmed with a pregnancy test.

Pregnancy is divided into three trimesters, each lasting for approximately 3 months. The first trimester includes conception, which is when the sperm fertilizes the egg. The fertilized egg then travels down the Fallopian tube and attaches to the inside of the uterus, where it begins to form the embryo and placenta. During the first trimester, the possibility of miscarriage (natural death of embryo or fetus) is at its highest. Around the middle of the second trimester, movement of the fetus may be felt. At 28 weeks, more than 90% of babies can survive outside of the uterus if provided with high-quality medical care, though babies born at this time will likely experience serious health complications such as heart and respiratory problems and long-term intellectual and developmental disabilities.

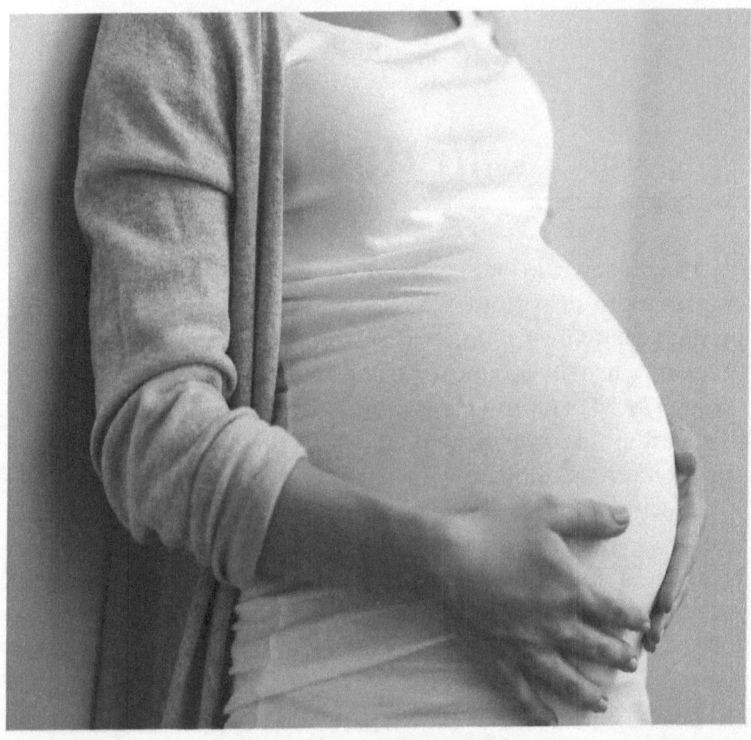

Prenatal care improves pregnancy outcomes. Prenatal care may include taking extra folic acid, avoiding drugs, tobacco smoking, and alcohol, taking regular exercise, having blood tests, and regular physical examinations. Complications of pregnancy may include disorders of high blood pressure, gestational diabetes, iron-deficiency anemia, and severe nausea and vomiting. In the ideal childbirth labor begins on its own when a woman is "at term". Babies born before 37 weeks are "preterm" and at higher risk of health problems such as cerebral palsy. Babies born between weeks 37 and 39 are considered "early term" while those born between weeks 39 and 41 are considered "full term".

Babies born between weeks 41 and 42 weeks are considered "late term" while after 42 weeks they are considered "post term". Delivery before 39 weeks by labor induction or caesarean section is not recommended unless required for other medical reasons.

About 213 million pregnancies occurred in 2012, of which, 190 million (89%) were in the developing world and 23 million (11%) were in the developed world. The number of pregnancies in women aged between 15 and 44 is 133 per 1,000 women. About 10% to 15% of recognized pregnancies end in miscarriage. In 2016, complications of pregnancy resulted in 230,600 maternal deaths, down from 377,000 deaths in 1990. Common causes include bleeding, infections, hypertensive diseases of pregnancy, obstructed labor, miscarriage, abortion, or ectopic pregnancy. Globally, 44% of pregnancies are unplanned. Over half (56%) of unplanned pregnancies are aborted. Among unintended pregnancies in the United States, 60% of the women used birth control to some extent during the month pregnancy occurred.

Terminology

Associated terms for pregnancy are *gravid* and *parous*. *Gravidus* and *gravid* come from the Latin word meaning "heavy" and a pregnant female is sometimes referred to as a *gravida*. *Gravidity* refers to the number of times that a female has been pregnant. Similarly, the term *parity* is used for the number of times that a female carries a pregnancy to a viable stage. Twins and other multiple births are counted as one pregnancy and birth. A woman who has never been pregnant is referred to as a *nulligravida*. A woman who is (or has been only) pregnant for the first time is referred to as a *primigravida*, and a woman in subsequent pregnancies as a *multigravida* or as *multiparous*. Therefore, during a second pregnancy a woman would be described as *gravida 2, para 1* and upon live delivery as *gravida 2, para 2*. In-progress pregnancies, abortions, miscarriages and/or stillbirths account for parity values being less than the gravida number. In the case of a multiple birth the gravida number and parity value are increased by one only. Women who have never carried a pregnancy more than 20 weeks are referred to as *nulliparous*.

A pregnancy is considered *term* at 37 weeks of gestation. It is *preterm* if less than 37 weeks and *postterm* at or beyond 42 weeks of gestation. American College of Obstetricians and Gynecologists have recommended further division with *early term* 37 weeks up to 39 weeks, *full term* 39 weeks up to 41 weeks, and *late term* 41 weeks up to 42 weeks. The terms *preterm* and *postterm* have largely replaced earlier terms of *premature* and *postmature*. *Preterm* and *postterm* are defined above, whereas *premature* and *postmature* have historical meaning and relate more to the infant's size and state of development rather than to the stage of pregnancy.

SIGNS AND SYMPTOMS

The usual signs and symptoms of pregnancy do not significantly interfere with activities of daily living or pose a health-threat to the mother or baby. However, pregnancy complications can cause other more severe symptoms, such as those associated with anemia.

Common signs and symptoms of pregnancy include:

- Tiredness
- Morning sickness
- Constipation
- Pelvic girdle pain
- Back pain
- Braxton Hicks contractions. Occasional, irregular, and often painless contractions that occur several times per day.
- Peripheral edema swelling of the lower limbs. Common complaint in advancing pregnancy. Can be caused by inferior vena cava syndrome resulting from compression of the inferior vena cava and pelvic veins by the uterus leading to increased hydrostatic pressure in lower extremities.
- Low blood pressure often caused by compression of both the inferior vena cava and the abdominal aorta (aortocaval compression syndrome).

- Increased urinary frequency. A common complaint, caused by increased intravascular volume, elevated glomerular filtration rate, and compression of the bladder by the expanding uterus.
- Urinary tract infection
- Varicose veins. Common complaint caused by relaxation of the venous smooth muscle and increased intravascular pressure.
- Hemorrhoids (piles). Swollen veins at or inside the anal area. Caused by impaired venous return, straining associated with constipation, or increased intra-abdominal pressure in later pregnancy.
- Regurgitation, heartburn, and nausea.
- Stretch marks
- Breast tenderness is common during the first trimester, and is more common in women who are pregnant at a young age.
- Melasma, also known as the mask of pregnancy, is a discoloration, most often of the face. It usually begins to fade several months after giving birth.

TIMELINE

The chronology of pregnancy is, unless otherwise specified, generally given as gestational age, where the starting point is the beginning of the woman's last menstrual period (LMP), or the corresponding age of the gestation as estimated by a more accurate method if available. Sometimes, timing may also use the fertilization age which is the age of the embryo.

Start of gestational age

The American Congress of Obstetricians and Gynecologists recommend the following methods to calculate gestational age:

- Directly calculating the days since the beginning of the last menstrual period.
- Early obstetric ultrasound, comparing the size of an embryo or fetus to that of a reference group of pregnancies

of known gestational age (such as calculated from last menstrual periods), and using the mean gestational age of other embryos or fetuses of the same size. If the gestational age as calculated from an early ultrasound is contradictory to the one calculated directly from the last menstrual period, it is still the one from the early ultrasound that is used for the rest of the pregnancy.

- In case of in vitro fertilization, calculating days since oocyte retrieval or co-incubation and adding 14 days.

Trimesters

Pregnancy is divided into three trimesters, each lasting for approximately 3 months. The exact length of each trimester can vary between sources.

- The first trimester begins with the start of gestational age as described above, that is, the beginning of week 1, or 0 weeks + 0 days of gestational age (GA). It ends at week 12 (11 weeks + 6 days of GA) or end of week 14 (13 weeks + 6 days of GA).
- The second trimester is defined as starting, between the beginning of week 13 (12 weeks +0 days of GA) and beginning of week 15 (14 weeks + 0 days of GA). It ends at the end of week 27 (26 weeks + 6 days of GA) or end of week 28 (27 weeks + 6 days of GA).
- The third trimester is defined as starting, between the beginning of week 28 (27 weeks + 0 days of GA) or beginning of week 29 (28 weeks + 0 days of GA). It lasts until childbirth.

Estimation of due date

Due date estimation basically follows two steps:

- Determination of which time point is to be used as origin for gestational age, as described in the section above.
- Adding the estimated gestational age at childbirth to the above time point. Childbirth on average occurs at a gestational age of 280 days (40 weeks), which is therefore often used as a standard estimation for individual

pregnancies. However, alternative durations as well as more individualized methods have also been suggested.

Naegele's rule is a standard way of calculating the due date for a pregnancy when assuming a gestational age of 280 days at childbirth. The rule estimates the expected date of delivery (EDD) by adding a year, subtracting three months, and adding seven days to the origin of gestational age. Alternatively there are mobile apps, which essentially always give consistent estimations compared to each other and correct for leap year, while pregnancy wheels made of paper can differ from each other by 7 days and generally do not correct for leap year.

Furthermore, actual childbirth has only a certain probability of occurring within the limits of the estimated due date. A study of singleton live births came to the result that childbirth has a standard deviation of 14 days when gestational age is estimated by first trimester ultrasound, and 16 days when estimated directly by last menstrual period.

DIAGNOSIS

The beginning of pregnancy may be detected either based on symptoms by the woman herself, or by using pregnancy tests. However, an important condition with serious health implications that is quite common is the denial of pregnancy by the pregnant woman. About one in 475 denials will last until around the 20th week of pregnancy. The proportion of cases of denial, persisting until delivery is about 1 in 2500. Conversely, some non-pregnant women have a very strong belief that they are pregnant along with some of the physical changes. This condition is known as a false pregnancy.

Physical signs

Most pregnant women experience a number of symptoms, which can signify pregnancy. A number of early medical signs are associated with pregnancy. These signs include:

- the presence of human chorionic gonadotropin (hCG) in the blood and urine

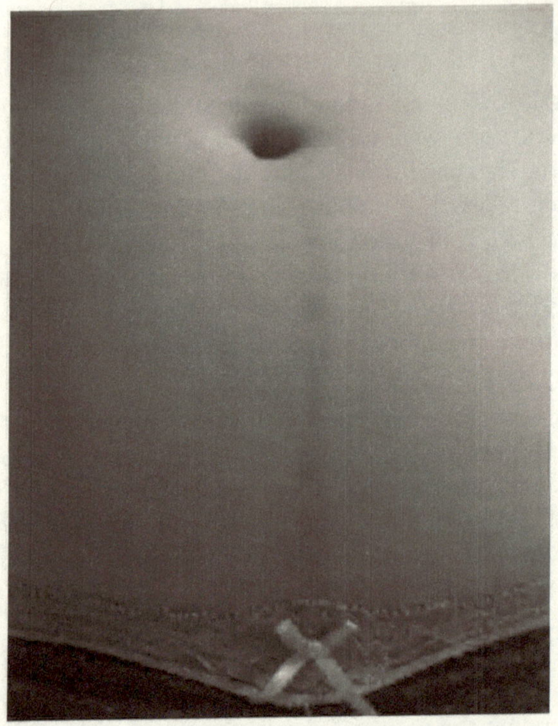

Linea nigra in a woman at 22 weeks pregnant.

- missed menstrual period
- implantation bleeding that occurs at implantation of the embryo in the uterus during the third or fourth week after last menstrual period
- increased basal body temperature sustained for over 2 weeks after ovulation
- Chadwick's sign (darkening of the cervix, vagina, and vulva)
- Goodell's sign (softening of the vaginal portion of the cervix)
- Hegar's sign (softening of the uterus isthmus)
- Pigmentation of the linea alba – linea nigra, (darkening of the skin in a midline of the abdomen, caused by hyperpigmentation resulting from hormonal changes, usually appearing around the middle of pregnancy).

- Darkening of the nipples and areolas due to an increase in hormones.

Biomarkers

Pregnancy detection can be accomplished using one or more various pregnancy tests, which detect hormones generated by the newly formed placenta, serving as biomarkers of pregnancy. Blood and urine tests can detect pregnancy 12 days after implantation. Blood pregnancy tests are more sensitive than urine tests (giving fewer false negatives). Home pregnancy tests are urine tests, and normally detect a pregnancy 12 to 15 days after fertilization. A quantitative blood test can determine approximately the date the embryo was conceived because hCG doubles every 36 to 48 hours. A single test of progesterone levels can also help determine how likely a fetus will survive in those with a threatened miscarriage (bleeding in early pregnancy).

Ultrasound

Obstetric ultrasonography can detect fetal abnormalities, detect multiple pregnancies, and improve gestational dating at 24 weeks. The resultant estimated gestational age and due date of the fetus are slightly more accurate than methods based on last menstrual period. Ultrasound is used to measure the nuchal fold in order to screen for Down syndrome.

MANAGEMENT

Prenatal care

Pre-conception counseling is care that is provided to a woman or couple to discuss conception, pregnancy, current health issues and recommendations for the period before pregnancy.

Prenatal medical care is the medical and nursing care recommended for women during pregnancy, time intervals and exact goals of each visit differ by country. Women who are high risk have better outcomes if they are seen regularly and frequently by a medical professional than women who are low risk. A woman can be labeled as high risk for different reasons including previous complications in pregnancy, complications in the current pregnancy, current medical diseases, or social issues.

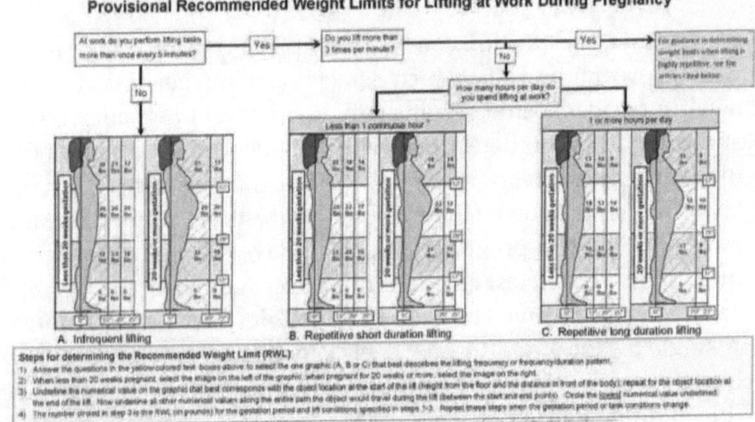

Flowchart showing the recommended weight limits for lifting at work during pregnancy as a function of lifting frequency, weeks of gestation, and the position of the lifted object relative to the lifter's body.

The aim of good prenatal care is prevention, early identification, and treatment of any medical complications. A basic prenatal visit consists of measurement of blood pressure, fundal height, weight and fetal heart rate, checking for symptoms of labor, and guidance for what to expect next.

Nutrition

Nutrition during pregnancy is important to ensure healthy growth of the fetus. Nutrition during pregnancy is different from the non-pregnant state. There are increased energy requirements and specific micronutrient requirements. Women benefit from education to encourage a balanced energy and protein intake during pregnancy. Some women may need professional medical advice if their diet is affected by medical conditions, food allergies, or specific religious/ ethical beliefs. Further studies are needed to access the effect of dietary advice to prevent gestational diabetes, although low quality evidence suggests some benefit.

Adequate periconceptional (time before and right after conception) folic acid (also called folate or Vitamin B_9) intake has been shown to decrease the risk of fetal neural tube defects, such as spina bifida. The neural tube develops during the first 28 days of pregnancy, a urine pregnancy test is not usually positive until 14 days post-conception, explaining the necessity to guarantee adequate folate intake before conception. Folate is abundant in green leafy vegetables, legumes, and citrus. In the United States and Canada, most wheat products (flour, noodles) are fortified with folic acid.

DHA omega-3 is a major structural fatty acid in the brain and retina, and is naturally found in breast milk. It is important for the woman to consume adequate amounts of DHA during pregnancy and while nursing to support her well-being and the health of her infant. Developing infants cannot produce DHA efficiently, and must receive this vital nutrient from the woman through the placenta during pregnancy and in breast milk after birth.

Several micronutrients are important for the health of the developing fetus, especially in areas of the world where insufficient nutrition is common. Women living in low and middle income countries are suggested to take multiple micronutrient supplements containing iron and folic acid. These supplements have been shown to improve birth outcomes in developing countries, but do not have an effect on perinatal mortality. Adequate intake of folic acid, and iron is often recommended. In developed areas, such as Western Europe and the United States, certain nutrients such as Vitamin D and calcium, required for bone development, may also require supplementation. Vitamin E supplementation has not been shown to improve birth outcomes. In a Cochrane review updated in 2021 there was insufficient evidence to support zinc supplementation to improve maternal or neonatal outcomes. Daily iron supplementation reduces the risk of maternal anemia. Studies of routine daily iron supplementation for pregnant women found improvement in blood iron levels, without a clear clinical benefit. The nutritional needs for women carrying twins or triplets are higher than those of women carrying one baby.

Women are counseled to avoid certain foods, because of the possibility of contamination with bacteria or parasites that can cause illness. Careful washing of fruits and raw vegetables may remove these pathogens, as may thoroughly cooking leftovers, meat, or processed meat. Unpasteurized dairy and deli meats may contain *Listeria,* which can cause neonatal meningitis, stillbirth and miscarriage. Pregnant women are also more prone to *Salmonella* infections, can be in eggs and poultry, which should be thoroughly cooked. Cat feces and undercooked meats may contain the parasite Toxoplasma gondii and can cause toxoplasmosis. Practicing good hygiene in the kitchen can reduce these risks.

Women are also counseled to eat seafood in moderation and to eliminate seafood known to be high in mercury because of the risk of birth defects. Pregnant women are counseled to consume caffeine in moderation, because large amounts of caffeine are associated with miscarriage. However, the relationship between caffeine, birthweight, and preterm birth is unclear.

Weight gain

The amount of healthy weight gain during a pregnancy varies. Weight gain is related to the weight of the baby, the placenta, extra circulatory fluid, larger tissues, and fat and protein stores. Most needed weight gain occurs later in pregnancy.

The Institute of Medicine recommends an overall pregnancy weight gain for those of normal weight (body mass index of 18.5–24.9), of 11.3–15.9 kg (25–35 pounds) having a singleton pregnancy. Women who are underweight (BMI of less than 18.5), should gain between 12.7 and 18 kg (28–40 lb), while those who are overweight (BMI of 25–29.9) are advised to gain between 6.8 and 11.3 kg (15–25 lb) and those who are obese (BMI e" 30) should gain between 5–9 kg (11–20 lb). These values reference the expectations for a term pregnancy.

During pregnancy, insufficient or excessive weight gain can compromise the health of the mother and fetus. The most effective intervention for weight gain in underweight women is not clear. Being or becoming overweight in pregnancy increases the risk of complications for mother and fetus, including cesarean section, gestational hypertension, pre-eclampsia, macrosomia and shoulder dystocia. Excessive weight gain can make losing weight after the pregnancy difficult. Some of these complications are risk factors for stroke.

Around 50% of women of childbearing age in developed countries like the United Kingdom are overweight or obese before pregnancy. Diet modification is the most effective way to reduce weight gain and associated risks in pregnancy.

Medication

Drugs used during pregnancy can have temporary or permanent effects on the fetus. Anything (including drugs) that can cause permanent deformities in the fetus are labeled as teratogens. In the U.S., drugs were classified into categories A, B, C, D and X based on the Food and Drug Administration (FDA) rating system to provide therapeutic guidance based on potential benefits and fetal risks. Drugs, including some multivitamins, that have demonstrated no fetal risks after controlled studies in humans are classified as Category A. On the other hand, drugs like thalidomide with proven fetal risks that outweigh all benefits are classified as Category X.

Recreational drugs

The use of recreational drugs in pregnancy can cause various pregnancy complications.

- Ethanol (the distinguishing ingredient of alcoholic drinks) consumed during pregnancy can cause one or more fetal alcohol spectrum disorders. According to the CDC, there is no known safe amount of alcohol during pregnancy and no safe time to drink during pregnancy, including before a woman knows that she is pregnant.

- Tobacco smoking during pregnancy can cause a wide range of behavioral, neurological, and physical difficulties. Smoking during pregnancy causes twice the risk of premature rupture of membranes, placental abruption and placenta previa. Smoking is associated with 30% higher odds of preterm birth.

- Prenatal cocaine exposure is associated with premature birth, birth defects and attention deficit disorder.
- Prenatal methamphetamine exposure can cause premature birth and congenital abnormalities. Short-term neonatal outcomes in methamphetamine babies show small deficits in infant neurobehavioral function and growth restriction. Long-term effects in terms of impaired brain development may also be caused by methamphetamine use.
- Cannabis in pregnancy has been shown to be teratogenic in large doses in animals, but has not shown any teratogenic effects in humans.

Exposure to toxins

Intrauterine exposure to environmental toxins in pregnancy has the potential to cause adverse effects on prenatal development, and to cause pregnancy complications. Air pollution has been associated with low birth weight infants. Conditions of particular severity in pregnancy include mercury poisoning and lead poisoning. To minimize exposure to environmental toxins, the *American College of Nurse-Midwives* recommends: checking whether the home has lead paint, washing all fresh fruits and vegetables thoroughly and buying organic produce, and avoiding cleaning products labeled "toxic" or any product with a warning on the label.

Pregnant women can also be exposed to toxins in the workplace, including airborne particles. The effects of wearing N95 filtering facepiece respirators are similar for pregnant women as for non-pregnant women, and wearing a respirator for one hour does not affect the fetal heart rate.

Sexual activity

Most women can continue to engage in sexual activity, including sexual intercourse, throughout pregnancy. Most research suggests that during pregnancy both sexual desire and frequency of sexual relations decrease. In context of this overall decrease in desire, some studies indicate a second-trimester increase, preceding a decrease during the third trimester.

Sex during pregnancy is a low-risk behavior except when the healthcare provider advises that sexual intercourse be avoided for particular medical reasons. For a healthy pregnant woman, there is no single *safe* or *right* way to have sex during pregnancy. Pregnancy alters the vaginal flora with a reduction in microscopic species/genus diversity.

Exercise

Regular aerobic exercise during pregnancy appears to improve (or maintain) physical fitness. Physical exercise during pregnancy appears to decrease the need for C-section, and even vigorous exercise carries no significant risks to babies and provides significant health benefits to the mother. Bed rest, outside of research studies, is not recommended as there is no evidence of benefit and potential harm.

The Clinical Practice Obstetrics Committee of Canada recommends that "All women without contraindications should be encouraged to participate in aerobic and strength-conditioning exercises as part of a healthy lifestyle during their pregnancy". Although an upper level of safe exercise intensity has not been established, women who were regular exercisers before pregnancy and who have uncomplicated pregnancies should be able to engage in high intensity exercise programs, without a higher risk of prematurity, lower birth weight, or gestational weight gain. In general, participation in a wide range of recreational activities appears to be safe, with the avoidance of those with a high risk of falling such as horseback riding or skiing or those that carry a risk of abdominal trauma, such as soccer or hockey.

The American College of Obstetricians and Gynecologists reports that in the past, the main concerns of exercise in pregnancy were focused on the fetus and any potential maternal benefit was thought to be offset by potential risks to the fetus. However, they write that more recent information suggests that in the uncomplicated pregnancy, fetal injuries are highly unlikely. They do, however, list several circumstances when a woman should contact her healthcare provider before continuing with an exercise program: vaginal bleeding, dyspnea before exertion, dizziness, headache, chest pain, muscle weakness, preterm labor, decreased fetal movement, amniotic fluid leakage, and calf pain or swelling (to rule out thrombophlebitis).

Sleep

It has been suggested that shift work and exposure to bright light at night should be avoided at least during the last trimester of pregnancy to decrease the risk of psychological and behavioral problems in the newborn.

Dental care

The increased levels of progesterone and estrogen during pregnancy make gingivitis more likely; the gums become edematous, red in colour, and tend to bleed.

Also a pyogenic granuloma or "pregnancy tumor", is commonly seen on the labial surface of the papilla. Lesions can be treated by local debridement or deep incision depending on their size, and by following adequate oral hygiene measures.

There have been suggestions that severe periodontitis may increase the risk of having preterm birth and low birth weight; however, a Cochrane review found insufficient evidence to determine if periodontitis can develop adverse birth outcomes.

Flying

In low risk pregnancies, most health care providers approve flying until about 36 weeks of gestational age. Most airlines allow pregnant women to fly short distances at less than 36 weeks, and long distances at less than 32 weeks. Many airlines require a doctor's note that approves flying, specially at over 28 weeks. During flights, the risk of deep vein thrombosis is decreased by getting up and walking occasionally, as well as by avoiding dehydration.

Full body scanners do not use ionizing radiation, and are safe in pregnancy. Airports can also possibly use backscatter X-ray scanners, which use a very low dose, but where safety in pregnancy is not fully established.

Microgravity

Since humans have gone to space the possibility of a pregnant person in space has been a possibility, though it is not supported by space agencies.

DISEASES IN PREGNANCY

A pregnant woman may have a pre-existing disease, which is not directly caused by the pregnancy, but may cause complications to develop that include a potential risk to the pregnancy; or a disease may develop during pregnancy.

- Diabetes mellitus and pregnancy deals with the interactions of diabetes mellitus (not restricted to gestational diabetes) and pregnancy. Risks for the child include miscarriage, growth restriction, growth acceleration, large for gestational age (macrosomia), polyhydramnios (too much amniotic fluid), and birth defects.

- Thyroid disease in pregnancy can, if uncorrected, cause adverse effects on fetal and maternal well-being. The deleterious effects of thyroid dysfunction can also extend beyond pregnancy and delivery to affect neurointellectual development in the early life of the child. Demand for thyroid hormones is increased during pregnancy, which may cause a previously unnoticed thyroid disorder to worsen.

- Untreated celiac disease can cause a miscarriage, intrauterine growth restriction, small for gestational age, low birthweight and preterm birth. Often reproductive disorders are the only manifestation of undiagnosed celiac disease and most cases are not recognized. Complications or failures of pregnancy cannot be explained simply by malabsorption, but by the autoimmune response elicited by the exposure to gluten, which causes damage to the placenta. The gluten-free diet avoids or reduces the risk of developing reproductive disorders in pregnant women with celiac disease. Also, pregnancy can be a trigger for the development of celiac disease in genetically susceptible women who are consuming gluten.

- Lupus in pregnancy confers an increased rate of fetal death *in utero,* miscarriage, and of neonatal lupus.
- Hypercoagulability in pregnancy is the propensity of pregnant women to develop thrombosis (blood clots). Pregnancy itself is a factor of hypercoagulability (pregnancy-induced hypercoagulability), as a physiologically adaptive mechanism to prevent postpartum bleeding. However, in combination with an underlying hypercoagulable state, the risk of thrombosis or embolism may become substantial.

MEDICAL IMAGING

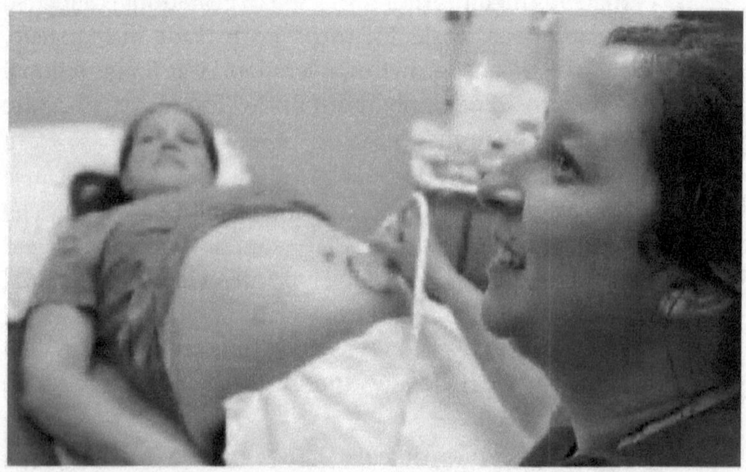

A pregnant woman undergoing an ultrasound. Ultrasound is used to check on the growth and development of the fetus.

Medical imaging may be indicated in pregnancy because of pregnancy complications, disease, or routine prenatal care. Medical ultrasonography including obstetric ultrasonography, and magnetic resonance imaging (MRI) without contrast agents are not associated with any risk for the mother or the fetus, and are the imaging techniques of choice for pregnant women. Projectional radiography, CT scan and nuclear medicine imaging result in some degree of ionizing radiation exposure, but in most cases the absorbed doses are not associated with harm to the baby.

At higher dosages, effects can include miscarriage, birth defects and intellectual disability.

Epidemiology

About 213 million pregnancies occurred in 2012 of which 190 million were in the developing world and 23 million were in the developed world. This is about 133 pregnancies per 1,000 women aged 15 to 44. About 10% to 15% of recognized pregnancies end in miscarriage. Globally, 44% of pregnancies are unplanned. Over half (56%) of unplanned pregnancies are aborted. In countries where abortion is prohibited, or only carried out in circumstances where the mother's life is at risk, 48% of unplanned pregnancies are aborted illegally. Compared to the rate in countries where abortion is legal, at 69%.

Of pregnancies in 2012, 120 million occurred in Asia, 54 million in Africa, 19 million in Europe, 18 million in Latin America and the Caribbean, 7 million in North America, and 1 million in Oceania. Pregnancy rates are 140 per 1000 women of childbearing age in the developing world and 94 per 1000 in the developed world.

The rate of pregnancy, as well as the ages at which it occurs, differ by country and region. It is influenced by a number of factors, such as cultural, social and religious norms; access to contraception; and rates of education. The total fertility rate (TFR) in 2013 was estimated to be highest in Niger (7.03 children/woman) and lowest in Singapore (0.79 children/woman).

In Europe, the average childbearing age has been rising continuously for some time. In Western, Northern, and Southern Europe, first-time mothers are on average 26 to 29 years old, up from 23 to 25 years at the start of the 1970s. In a number of European countries (Spain), the mean age of women at first childbirth has crossed the 30-year threshold.

This process is not restricted to Europe. Asia, Japan and the United States are all seeing average age at first birth on the rise, and increasingly the process is spreading to countries in the developing world like China, Turkey and Iran. In the US, the average age of first childbirth was 25.4 in 2010.

In the United States and United Kingdom, 40% of pregnancies are unplanned, and between a quarter and half of those unplanned pregnancies were unwanted pregnancies.

SOCIETY AND CULTURE

In most cultures, pregnant women have a special status in society and receive particularly gentle care. At the same time, they are subject to expectations that may exert great psychological pressure, such as having to produce a son and heir. In many traditional societies, pregnancy must be preceded by marriage, on pain of ostracism of mother and (illegitimate) child.

Overall, pregnancy is accompanied by numerous customs that are often subject to ethnological research, often rooted in traditional medicine or religion. The baby shower is an example of a modern custom.

Pregnancy is an important topic in sociology of the family. The prospective child may preliminarily be placed into numerous social roles. The parents' relationship and the relation between parents and their surroundings are also affected.

A belly cast may be made during pregnancy as a keepsake.

Arts

Images of pregnant women, especially small figurines, were made in traditional cultures in many places and periods, though it is rarely one of the most common types of image. These include ceramic figures from some Pre-Columbian cultures, and a few figures from most of the ancient Mediterranean cultures. Many of these seem to be connected with fertility. Identifying whether such figures are actually meant to show pregnancy is often a problem, as well as understanding their role in the culture concerned.

Among the oldest surviving examples of the depiction of pregnancy are prehistoric figurines found across much of Eurasia and collectively known as Venus figurines. Some of these appear to be pregnant.

Due to the important role of the Mother of God in Christianity, the Western visual arts have a long tradition of depictions of pregnancy, especially in the biblical scene of the Visitation, and devotional images called a *Madonna del Parto*.

The unhappy scene usually called *Diana and Callisto*, showing the moment of discovery of Callisto's forbidden pregnancy, is sometimes painted from the Renaissance onwards. Gradually, portraits of pregnant women began to appear, with a particular fashion for "pregnancy portraits" in elite portraiture of the years around 1600.

Pregnancy, and especially pregnancy of unmarried women, is also an important motif in literature. Notable examples include Hardy's *Tess of the d'Urbervilles* and Goethe's *Faust*.

Infertility

Modern reproductive medicine offers many forms of assisted reproductive technology for couples who stay childless against their will, such as fertility medication, artificial insemination, *in vitro* fertilization and surrogacy.

Abortion

An abortion is the termination of an embryo or fetus, either naturally or via medical methods. When carried out by choice, it is usually within the first trimester, sometimes in the second, and rarely in the third.

Not using contraception, contraceptive failure, poor family planning or rape can lead to undesired pregnancies. Legality of socially indicated abortions varies widely both internationally and through time.

In most countries of Western Europe, abortions during the first trimester were a criminal offense a few decades ago but have since been legalized, sometimes subject to mandatory consultations. In Germany, for example, as of 2009 less than 3% of abortions had a medical indication.

Legal protection

Many countries have various legal regulations in place to protect pregnant women and their children. Maternity Protection

Convention ensures that pregnant women are exempt from activities such as night shifts or carrying heavy stocks.

Maternity leave typically provides paid leave from work during roughly the last trimester of pregnancy and for some time after birth. Notable extreme cases include Norway (8 months with full pay) and the United States (no paid leave at all except in some states). Moreover, many countries have laws against pregnancy discrimination.

In the United States, some actions that result in miscarriage or stillbirth are considered crimes. One law that does so is the federal Unborn Victims of Violence Act. In 2014, the American state of Tennessee passed a law which allows prosecutors to charge a woman with criminal assault if she uses illegal drugs during her pregnancy and her fetus or newborn is considered harmed as a result.

2

Symptoms of Pregnancy

You may notice some signs and symptoms before you even take a pregnancy test. Others will appear weeks later, as your hormone levels change.

EARLY PREGNANCY SYMPTOMS

Early signs and symptoms of pregnancy: Things you might notice before you start prenatal care.

Could you be pregnant? Before you test, read this list of classic clues.

Are you pregnant? The proof is really in the pregnancy test. But you may suspect — or hope — that you're expecting, even before you miss a period, if you experience one or more of the following signs and symptoms of pregnancy. These early clues may begin in the first few weeks after conception.

Tender, swollen breasts or nipples

One of the first physical changes of pregnancy is a change in the way your breasts feel. They may feel tender, tingly or sore. Or they may feel fuller and heavier. As early as two weeks after conception, your breasts start to grow and change in preparation for producing milk. The primary cause of these changes is increased production of the hormones estrogen and progesterone. Changes in your breasts are often most dramatic when you're pregnant for the first time.

Fatigue

Many women feel wiped out during pregnancy, especially in the early stages. This may be nature's way of persuading moms-to-be to take extra naps, in preparation for the sleepless nights ahead. But there's also a physical reason for fatigue.

During the early weeks of pregnancy, your body is working hard — pumping out hormones and producing more blood to carry nutrients to your baby. To accommodate this increased blood flow, your heart pumps harder and faster. Plus, progesterone is a natural central nervous system depressant, so high levels of this hormone may make you sleepy. In addition, the possibility of pregnancy can bring about a range of feelings and concerns that may sap your energy and disturb sleep.

Slight bleeding or cramping

Some women experience a small amount of spotting or bleeding very early in pregnancy, about 10 to 14 days after fertilization. Known as implantation bleeding, it happens when the fertilized egg first attaches to the lining of the uterus. This type of bleeding is usually a bit earlier, spottier and lighter in colour than a usual period and doesn't last long.

Many women also experience cramping very early in pregnancy as the uterus begins to enlarge. These cramps are similar to menstrual cramps.

Nausea with or without vomiting

Morning sickness is one of the telltale signs of early pregnancy. Most women feel some sickness around four to eight weeks of pregnancy, but the queasiness can begin as early as two weeks after conception.

Although nausea and vomiting during pregnancy is commonly called morning sickness, it can occur at any time of the day. It seems to stem from the rapidly rising levels of estrogen produced by the placenta and the fetus. These hormones cause the stomach to empty somewhat more slowly, which could be part of the problem. Pregnant women also have a heightened sense of smell, so a variety of odors — such as foods cooking, coffee, perfume or cigarette smoke — can trigger nausea.

Food aversions or cravings

Turning up your nose at certain foods is often the first hint that you're pregnant. Even the smell of some foods may cause a wave of nausea in early pregnancy. One study suggests that pregnant women experience a unique aversion to coffee in the early weeks of pregnancy. Meat, dairy products and spicy foods are other common objects of repulsion.

Food cravings are common, too. Like most other symptoms of pregnancy, these food preferences can be chalked up to hormonal changes. Pregnant women typically find that their food tastes change somewhat, especially in the first trimester, when hormones have the strongest impact.

Frequent urination

Many pregnant women find themselves running to the bathroom more often than usual. During the first trimester of pregnancy, this is caused by the enlarging uterus pushing on your bladder.

Headaches

If you're pregnant, you may be troubled by frequent, mild headaches. Early in pregnancy, headaches may be the result of increased blood circulation caused by hormonal changes.

Constipation

Constipation is another common early indication of pregnancy. An increase in progesterone causes digestion to slow down, so food passes more slowly through the gastrointestinal tract, which can lead to constipation.

Mood swings

You're a no-nonsense kind of woman — so what's with this crying over Hallmark commercials ? The flood of hormones in your body in early pregnancy can make you unusually emotional and weepy. Swings in your mood, from bliss to deep gloom, also are common, especially in the first trimester.

Faintness and dizziness

It's common for pregnant women to be lightheaded or dizzy. These sensations usually result from circulatory changes as your blood vessels dilate and your blood pressure drops. Early in pregnancy, faint feelings may also be triggered by low blood sugar.

Raised basal body temperature

Your basal body temperature (BBT) is your oral temperature when you first wake up in the morning. This temperature spikes slightly soon after ovulation and remains at that level until your next period. If you've been charting your BBT to determine when you ovulate, its continued elevation for more than two weeks may mean you're pregnant. In fact, BBT stays elevated throughout your pregnancy.

Are you really pregnant?

Unfortunately, these signs and symptoms aren't unique to pregnancy. Some can indicate that you're getting sick or that your period is about to start. And, conversely, you can be pregnant without ever experiencing these symptoms. Still, if you notice any of the tip-offs on this list, make plans to take a home pregnancy test, especially if you're not keeping track of your menstrual cycle or if it varies widely from one month to the next. Also take extra good care of yourself. You just might be taking care for two.

Home pregnancy tests: Useful products with some drawbacks

Are you feeling nauseated or fatigued? Is your period late? If so, taking a home pregnancy test may be a reasonable next step.

Whether it's your first time or your fifth time, taking a home pregnancy test (HPT) can be nerve-racking. To quell your anxiety, find out how HPTs work, what can affect the results and when to visit the doctor.

How HPTs detect pregnancy

As soon as a fertilized egg is implanted in your uterus, your body starts releasing a hormone called human chorionic gonadotropin (HCG) into your bloodstream. Your blood and urine contain HCG throughout pregnancy. If a test detects HCG in your blood or urine, it almost always means you're pregnant.

All HPTs check for HCG in the urine instead of the blood. The tests come in these three types:

- *The dipstick test:* This type of HPT requires that you either place the end of the dipstick in your urine stream as you urinate or immerse the dipstick in a container of collected urine for five to ten seconds. A minute or two later, the result will appear on the strip as a symbol (such as a plus or minus sign), a line, a colour change or even the words *pregnant* or *not pregnant.*

- *The collection cup test:* For this test, you need a sample of urine collected midstream — a few seconds after you've started to urinate. When you have the sample, you take some of the urine into an eyedropper and squeeze five or six drops on a test disc provided in the HPT kit. The urine makes the disc change to a particular colour if you are pregnant and to a different colour if you aren't.

- *The chemical mixing test:* In this test, you place a small amount of urine in a test tube with a liquid or powder chemical mixture. If the chemicals make the urine change colour, it means you're pregnant.

Grocery stores and drugstores carry a wide variety of HPT kits. They're quick, easy to use and fairly inexpensive, with prices ranging from $7.99 to $19.99.

Most HPTs claim to be 97 percent to 99 percent accurate if they're used correctly. Instructions are slightly different from kit to kit, so read through them carefully before you start. Then, for the most accurate result, follow the instructions closely.

Results can be incorrect

Although HPTs are generally reliable, you have to use them

properly. Otherwise, you may get a false-positive or false-negative result. Possible causes of false-positives include:

- *Using an unclean urine collection cup:* If your HPT uses a cup, be sure that it's clean and free of any soap residue. Detergent buildup on the cup may cause a false-positive result.

- *Using an old or damaged kit:* Be sure to check the expiration date on the box before taking the test. Also, a kit that has been exposed to heat, dampness or vibration may have a false-positive result.

- *Having an impure urine sample:* Blood in your urine — from a urinary tract infection, for example — may lead to a false-positive result, as may protein, which sometimes gets into the urine if you have kidney damage. Certain rare tumors may also secrete HCG and cause a false-positive result.

- *Taking certain prescription drugs:* Certain medications such as anticonvulsants, anti-Parkinson drugs and tranquilisers may cause false-positive results. Also, diuretics (often used to treat high blood pressure) and promethazine (used to treat allergy symptoms and nausea) may trigger a false-positive result.

You may get a false-negative result from:

- *Taking the test too early.* Taking a pregnancy test too early may give you a negative result when you actually are pregnant. Hold off on the HPT until your period is at least one day late. That's the earliest an HPT can possibly detect pregnancy — in fact, most HPTs are unreliable until your period is a week late. The bottom line: If you have a negative HPT on the day after your period was due, wait a week. Then, if your period hasn't started, repeat the test.

- *Timing the test wrong:* Perform the test within 15 minutes of collecting the urine sample. After you start the test, be sure to give it time to work, but don't wait longer than the instructions tell you to. If you tend to lose track of minutes, use a timer or a clock.

- *Using diluted urine:* Consuming large amounts of fluid before taking an HPT may also cause a false-negative test result. It's best to take an HPT first thing in the morning because that's when your urine is the most concentrated.

If you have any questions about how to perform the test or interpret the results, look in the instructions for a toll-free help number to call. Also, since many pregnancy tests come in packages of two, don't hesitate to take a second test if your first test results are unclear.

When to contact the doctor?

As soon as you find out you're pregnant, it's time to make an appointment with your doctor or nurse practitioner to begin your prenatal care. At this point, your doctor or nurse may follow up with a blood test and pelvic exam to confirm your pregnancy. Blood tests can detect HCG as early as six to eight days after conception (when the egg is fertilized).

A blood test can also quantify the level of HCG in your blood, providing clues to the progress of your pregnancy. In typical pregnancies, HCG levels increase dramatically during the first trimester and decrease somewhat thereafter. An abnormal HCG level might be a sign of a problem, such as miscarriage or tubal pregnancy, or it might mean you are carrying more than one baby. If you have abnormal HCG levels, your doctor will address them and monitor you closely during your pregnancy. Unless there are other signs to cause concern, the HCG test is usually not performed more than once.

You should also talk to your doctor if you miss your period for more than two months and you're not pregnant. Pregnancy is not the only possible cause of irregular menstruation. Women using birth control pills, for example, often miss periods and think, incorrectly, that their contraceptive method has failed them. If you get a negative result on an HPT after missing a period while you're on the pill, continue to take it as directed. Talk to your doctor before discontinuing the pill if you're repeatedly missing periods.

Other things that can make you miss periods include:
- Breast-feeding
- Certain medications
- A serious illness
- Malnutrition or obesity
- Extreme exercise regimens
- Stress
- The onset of menopause

By talking with you about your lifestyle and health, your doctor will be able to recommend ways to get your menstrual cycle back on track.

MISSED PERIOD

A missed period is one of the earliest symptoms of pregnancy (and maybe the most classic one). However, a missed period doesn't necessarily mean you're pregnant, especially if your cycle tends to be irregular.

There are many health conditions other than pregnancy that can cause a late or missed period.

Headache

Headaches are common in early pregnancy. They're usually caused by altered hormone levels and increased blood volume. Contact your doctor if your headaches don't go away or are especially painful.

Spotting

Some women may experience light bleeding and spotting in early pregnancy. This bleeding is most often the result of implantation. Implantation usually occurs one to two weeks after fertilization.

Early pregnancy bleeding can also result from relatively minor conditions such as an infection or irritation. The latter often affects the surface of the cervix (which is very sensitive during pregnancy).

Bleeding can also sometimes signal a serious pregnancy complication, such as miscarriage, ectopic pregnancy, or placenta previa. Always contact your doctor if you're concerned.

Weight gain

You can expect to gain between 1 and 4 pounds in your first few months of pregnancy. Weight gain becomes more noticeable toward the beginning of your second trimester.

PREGNANCY-INDUCED HYPERTENSION

High blood pressure, or hypertension, sometimes develops during pregnancy. A number of factors can increase your risk, including:

- being overweight or obese
- smoking
- having a prior history or a family history of pregnancy-induced hypertension

Heartburn

Hormones released during pregnancy can sometimes relax the valve between your stomach and esophagus. When stomach acid leaks out, this can result in heartburn.

Constipation

Hormone changes during early pregnancy can slow down your digestive system. As a result, you may become constipated.

Cramps

As the muscles in your uterus begin to stretch and expand, you may feel a pulling sensation that resembles menstrual cramps. If spotting or bleeding occurs alongside your cramps, it could signal a miscarriage or an ectopic pregnancy.

Back pain

Hormones and stress on the muscles are the biggest causes of back pain in early pregnancy. Later on, your increased weight and shifted center of gravity may add to your back pain. Around half of all pregnant women report back pain during their pregnancy.

Anemia

Pregnant women have an increased risk of anemia, which causes symptoms such as lightheadedness and dizziness.

The condition can lead to premature birth and low birth weight. Prenatal care usually involves screening for anemia.

Depression

Between 14 and 23 percent of all pregnant women develop depression during their pregnancy. The many biological and emotional changes you experience can be contributing causes.

Be sure to tell your doctor if you don't feel like your usual self.

Insomnia

Insomnia is another common symptom of early pregnancy. Stress, physical discomfort, and hormonal changes can be contributing causes. A balanced diet, good sleep habits, and yoga stretches can all help you get a good night's sleep.

Breast changes

Breast changes are one of the first noticeable signs of pregnancy. Even before you're far enough along for a positive test, your breasts may begin to feel tender, swollen, and generally heavy or full. Your nipples may also become larger and more sensitive, and the areolae may darken.

Acne

Because of increased androgen hormones, many women experience acne in early pregnancy. These hormones can make your skin oilier, which can clog pores. Pregnancy acne is usually temporary and clears up after the baby is born.

Vomiting

Vomiting is a component of "morning sickness," a common symptom that usually appears within the first four months. Morning sickness is often the first sign that you're pregnant. Increased hormones during early pregnancy are the main cause.

Hip pain

Hip pain is common during pregnancy and tends to increase in late pregnancy. It can have a variety of causes, including:
- pressure on your ligaments
- sciatica
- changes in your posture
- a heavier uterus

Diarrhea

Diarrhea and other digestive difficulties occur frequently during pregnancy. Hormone changes, a different diet, and added stress are all possible explanations. If diarrhea lasts more than a few days, contact your doctor to make sure you don't become dehydrated.

STRESS AND PREGNANCY

While pregnancy is usually a happy time, it can also be a source of stress. A new baby means big changes to your body, your personal relationships, and even your finances. Don't hesitate to ask your doctor for help if you begin to feel overwhelmed.

PREGNANCY PREVENTION

Women who have male sexual partners should consider birth control if they're not interested in becoming pregnant. Some methods of pregnancy prevention work better for certain individuals. Talk to your doctor about birth control that's right for you. A few of the most common birth control methods are discussed below:

Birth control method	Effectiveness rate
Intrauterine devices (IUDs)	Over 99 percent
The pill	99 percent with perfect use; around 91 percent with typical use
Male condom	98 percent with perfect use; around 82 percentTrusted SourceTrusted Source with typical use
Female condom (or internal condom)	95 percent effective with perfect use; around 79 percent with typical use

| Morning-after pill | Up to 95 percent (taken within one day of sexual contact); 75 to 89 percent (taken within three days) |
| Natural family planning (NFP) | 75 percent when used on its own |

Intrauterine devices (IUDs)

Intrauterine devices (IUDs) work by mostly by stopping fertilization. They're currently the most effective form of birth control. The downside is that they don't prevent sexually transmitted diseases (STDs).

The pill and other hormonal birth control methods

Birth control pills, patches and the vaginal ring work by controlling the hormone levels in a woman's body. They're available by prescription.

Actions that can reduce the effectiveness of these methods include forgetting to use them as prescribed. Effectiveness rates that mention "typical use" account for these types of human errors.

Other forms of hormonal birth control include the patch and the vaginal ring. They're also available by prescription, and their effectiveness rates are similar to those of the pill.

Condoms and other barrier methods

Condoms, diaphragms, and sponges are convenient and inexpensive forms of birth control that can be bought without a prescription.

They're most effective when used correctly every time you have sexual intercourse. If you're relying on these barrier methods to avoid getting pregnant, also consider using an additional method of contraception such as spermicide or a birth control pill.

Other barrier methods include diaphragms and sponges. They can be bought without a prescription.

Emergency contraception

Several morning-after pills are available, both over the counter and by prescription. These pills aren't intended as regular forms of birth control. Instead, they can act as a backup if you have unprotected sex or forget to use your regular form of birth control.

They must be used within 120 hours (five days) of sexual contact to be effective. Some pills are most effective when taken within 72 hours (three days).

Natural family planning (NFP)

Natural family planning (NFP), or fertility awareness, is the birth control method with the highest failure rate. With NFP, a woman tracks her menstrual cycle so that she can predict when she'll ovulate. She'll then avoid intercourse during her fertile window.

Accidental pregnancies can occur because there are many variables affecting a woman's cycle from month to month.

PREGNANCY OR PMS

The symptoms of early pregnancy can often mimic those of premenstrual syndrome (PMS). It may be difficult for a woman to know if she's pregnant or simply experiencing the onset of another menstrual period.

It's important for a woman to know as soon as possible if she's pregnant so that she can get proper prenatal care. She may also want to make certain lifestyle changes, such as abstaining from alcohol, taking prenatal vitamins, and optimizing her diet.

Taking a pregnancy test is the best, and easiest, way to determine if it's PMS or early pregnancy. You can take a home test or visit your healthcare provider.

Some common symptoms of both PMS and early pregnancy include:

- breast pain
- bleeding
- mood changes
- fatigue
- food sensitivities
- cramping

Early pregnancy and PMS are often difficult to tell apart. Learn to distinguish between the two with the help of this Venn diagram.

PREGNANCY DIET

A healthy pregnancy diet should be much the same as your typical healthy diet, only with 340 to 450 additional calories per day. Aim for a healthy mix of foods, including:

- complex carbohydrates
- protein
- vegetables and fruits
- grains and legumes
- healthy fats

If you already eat a healthy diet, you'll only need to make slight changes. Fluids, fiber, and iron-rich foods are especially important during pregnancy.

Vitamins and minerals

Pregnant women require larger amounts of some vitamins and minerals than women who aren't pregnant. Folic acid and zinc are just two examples.

Once you find out you're pregnant, you may wish to increase your vitamin and mineral intake with the help of supplements. Be sure to read nutrition labels and seek your doctor's advice before using any supplements or over-the-counter (OTC) medications.

Although rare, taking supplements could result in vitamin toxicity or overdose. However, a complete prenatal vitamin will probably contain a good mix of the nutrients that you need for a healthy pregnancy.

PREGNANCY AND EXERCISE

Exercise is essential to keeping you fit, relaxed, and ready for labor. Yoga stretches in particular will help you stay limber. It's important not to overdo your stretches, however, as you could risk injury.

Other good exercises for pregnancy are gentle Pilates, walking, and swimming.

You may need to modify your current fitness routine to accommodate your changing body and lower energy levels. Work with your healthcare provider or a personal trainer to ensure that you aren't overexerting yourself. Get more ideas for staying fit in your first trimester.

PREGNANCY MASSAGE

Practicing relaxation techniques can help relieve some of the stress and anxiety you may feel throughout your pregnancy.

If you're searching for ways to stay calm, consider trying a prenatal massage. A prenatal massage is good for relieving mild tension. It may also help ease your body and muscle aches.

Massages are generally safe at any time during your pregnancy. Some facilities avoid performing them in the first trimester because the risk of miscarriage is highest during this period.

Getting your doctor's approval before you get a massage is a good idea, especially if you've had pain in your calves or other parts of your legs.

Essential oils

Using essential oils during pregnancy is controversial. Some healthcare professionals say that certain oils can be safe and helpful for relaxing and alleviating pain during pregnancy and labor. However, they also warn against using the oils in the first trimester.

According to the nonprofit National Association for Holistic Aromatherapy, the main point of contention is whether oils used during pregnancy can harm the growing baby if they cross over into the placenta.

More research is needed about using essential oils during pregnancy and labor. If you plan to use them, seek guidance from your healthcare provider.

WHEN TO SEEK MEDICAL CARE

Most women in their 20s or early 30s have a good chance of

a problem-free pregnancy. Teens and women over the age of 35 are at a higher risk for health complications.

Underlying conditions

Underlying health conditions such as high blood pressure, diabetes, or cardiovascular disease will increase your risk of pregnancy complications. Other examples include:

- cancer
- kidney disease
- epilepsy

If you have one of these conditions, ensure that it's properly monitored and treated throughout your pregnancy. Otherwise, it can lead to miscarriage, poor fetal growth, and birth defects.

Other risk factors

Other factors that can affect an otherwise healthy pregnancy include:

- multiple-birth pregnancies, such as twins or triplets
- infections, including STDs
- being overweight or obese
- anemia

Pregnancy complications

Pregnancy complications can involve the baby's health, the mother's health, or both. They can occur during pregnancy or delivery.

Common pregnancy complications include:

- high blood pressure
- gestational diabetes
- preeclampsia
- preterm labor
- miscarriage

Addressing them early can minimize the harms done to the mother or the baby. Know your options when it comes to treating pregnancy complications.

PREGNANCY AND LABOR

Sometime after your fourth month of pregnancy, you may begin to experience Braxton-Hicks contractions, or false labor. They're completely normal and serve to prepare your uterus for the job ahead of real labor.

Braxton-Hicks contractions don't occur at regular intervals, and they don't increase in intensity. If you experience regular contractions before week 37, it could be preterm labor. If this occurs, call your healthcare provider for help.

Early labor

Labor contractions are generally classified as early labor contractions and active labor contractions. Early labor contractions last between 30 and 45 seconds. They may be far apart at first, but by the end of early labor, contractions will be about five minutes apart.

Your water might break early during labor, or your doctor may break it for you later on during your labor. When the cervix begins to open, you'll see a blood-tinged discharge coating your mucous plug.

Active labor

In active labor, the cervix dilates, and the contractions get closer together and become more intense.

If you're in active labor, you should call your healthcare provider and head to your birth setting. If you're unsure whether it's active labor, it's still a good idea to call and check in.

Labor pain

Pain will be at its height during active labor. Have a discussion with your doctor about your preferred method of dealing with pain.

You may choose drug-free measures such as meditation, yoga, or listening to music.

If you choose to manage your pain with drugs, your doctor will need to know whether to use analgesics or anesthetics.

Analgesics, such as meperidine (Demerol), dull the pain but allow you to retain some feeling. Anesthetics, such as an epidural, prevent certain muscle movement and completely block the pain.

PROGNOSIS

You're likely to move through each week of your pregnancy without too much trouble. Pregnancy brings with it many changes to your body, but those changes don't always have a serious impact on your health.

However, certain lifestyle choices can either help or actively harm your baby's development.

Some actions that can keep you and your baby healthy include:
- taking a multivitamin
- getting sufficient sleep
- practicing safe sex
- getting a flu shot
- visiting your dentist

Some things you'll want to avoid include:
- smoking
- drinking alcohol
- eating raw meat, deli meat, or unpasteurized dairy products
- sitting in a hot tub or sauna
- gaining too much weight

Medications

It can be hard to determine which medications you can take during pregnancy and which ones you should avoid. You'll have to weigh the benefits to your health against potential risks to the developing baby.

Ask your healthcare provider about any drugs you may take, even OTC ones for minor ailments such as headaches.

According to the Food and Drug Administration (FDA)Trusted SourceTrusted Source, each year 50 percent of pregnant women in the United States report taking at least one medication.

In the 1970s, the FDA created a letter systemTrusted SourceTrusted Source to categorize drugs and their perceived risk to pregnant women. However, they began to phase out this letter system (and use updated drug labeling) in 2015. Their new rules for drug labelingTrusted SourceTrusted Source only apply to prescription drugs.

The service MotherToBaby also provides up-to-date information on the safety of specific drugs.

The takeaway

Under the Affordable Care Act (ACA), all health insurance plans in the United States are required to offer some level of prenatal care.

Once your pregnancy's been confirmed, call your insurance provider to get an idea of what's covered by your specific plan. If you don't have health insurance when you find out you're pregnant, speak to your doctor about steps you can take to get coverage.

The timing of your first prenatal visit may depend on your overall health. Most women may have their first visit during week 8 of pregnancy. Women whose pregnancies are considered high-risk, such as those who are over 35 or have chronic conditions, may be asked to see their doctors earlier.

There are many ways to mentally and physically prepare for labor. Many hospitals offer birthing classes prior to delivery so that women may better understand the signs and stages of labor.

In your third trimester, you may want to prepare a hospital bag of toiletries, sleepwear, and other everyday essentials. This bag would be ready to take with you when labor begins. During the third trimester, you and your doctor should also discuss your labor and delivery plan in detail.

Knowing when to go to the birth setting, who'll be assisting in the birth, and what role your doctor will play in the process can contribute to greater peace of mind as you enter those final weeks.

3

Duration of Pregnancy

There are, as a rule, 266 to 270 days between ovulation and childbirth, with extremes of 250 and 285 days. Physicians usually determine the date of the estimated time for delivery by adding seven days to the first day of the last menstrual period and counting forward nine calendar months; i.e., if the last period began on January 10, the date of delivery is October 17.

Courts of law, in determining the legitimacy of a child, may accept much shorter or much longer periods of gestation as being within the periods of possible duration of a pregnancy. One court in the state of New York has accepted a pregnancy of 355 days as legitimate.

British courts have recognized 331 and 346 days as legitimate with the approval of medical consultants. Fully developed infants have been born as early as 221 days after the first day of the mother's last menstrual period.

Because the exact date of ovulation is usually not known, it is seldom possible to make an accurate estimate of the date of delivery. There is a 5 percent chance that a baby will be born on the exact date estimated from the above rule. There is a 25 percent chance that it will be born within four days before or after the estimated date. There is a 50 percent chance that delivery will occur on the estimated date plus or minus seven days. There is a 95 percent chance that the baby will be born within plus or minus 14 days of the estimated date of delivery.

PREGNANCY - WEEK BY WEEK

- Pregnancy is counted as 40 weeks, starting from the first day of the mother's last menstrual period. Your estimated date to birth is only to give you a guide. Babies come when they are ready and you need to be patient.
- The gender and inherited characteristics of the baby are decided at the moment of conception.

The unborn baby spends around 38 weeks in the womb, but the average length of pregnancy (gestation) is counted as 40 weeks. This is because pregnancy is counted from the first day of the woman's last period, not the date of conception, which generally occurs two weeks later.

Pregnancy is divided into three trimesters:

- First trimester – conception to 12 weeks
- Second trimester – 12 to 24 weeks
- Third trimester – 24 to 40 weeks.

Conception

The moment of conception is when the woman's ovum (egg) is fertilised by the man's sperm. The gender and inherited characteristics are decided in that instant.

Week 1

This first week is actually your menstrual period. Because your expected birth date (EDD or EDB) is calculated from the first day of your last period, this week counts as part of your 40-week pregnancy, even though your baby hasn't been conceived yet.

Week 2

Fertilisation of your egg by the sperm will take place near the end of this week.

Week 3

Thirty hours after conception, the cell splits into two. Three days later, the cell (zygote) has divided into 16 cells. After two more days, the zygote has migrated from the fallopian tube to the uterus (womb). Seven days after conception, the zygote burrows itself into the plump uterine lining (endometrium). The zygote is now known as a blastocyst.

Week 4

The developing baby is tinier than a grain of rice. The rapidly dividing cells are in the process of forming the various body systems, including the digestive system.

Week 5

The evolving neural tube will eventually become the central nervous system (brain and spinal cord).

Week 6

The baby is now known as an embryo. It is around 3 mm in length. By this stage, it is secreting special hormones that prevent the mother from having a menstrual period.

Week 7

The heart is beating. The embryo has developed its placenta and amniotic sac. The placenta is burrowing into the uterine wall to access oxygen and nutrients from the mother's bloodstream.

Week 8

The embryo is now around 1.3 cm in length. The rapidly growing spinal cord looks like a tail. The head is disproportionately large.

Week 9

The eyes, mouth and tongue are forming. The tiny muscles allow the embryo to start moving about. Blood cells are being made by the embryo's liver.

Week 10

The embryo is now known as a fetus and is about 2.5 cm in length. All of the bodily organs are formed. The hands and feet, which previously looked like nubs or paddles, are now evolving fingers and toes. The brain is active and has brain waves.

Week 11

Teeth are budding inside the gums. The tiny heart is developing further.

Week 12

The fingers and toes are recognisable, but still stuck together with webs of skin. The first trimester combined screening test (maternal blood test + ultrasound of baby) can be done around this time. This test checks for trisomy 18 (Edward syndrome) and trisomy 21 (Down syndrome).

Week 13

The fetus can swim about quite vigorously. It is now more than 7 cm in length.

Week 14

The eyelids are fused over the fully developed eyes. The baby can now mutely cry, since it has vocal cords. It may even start sucking its thumb. The fingers and toes are growing nails.

Week 16

The fetus is around 14 cm in length. Eyelashes and eyebrows have appeared, and the tongue has tastebuds. The second trimester maternal serum screening will be offered at this time if the first trimester test was not done.

Week 18-20

An ultrasound will be offered. This fetal morphology scan is to check for structural abnormalities, position of placenta and multiple pregnancies. Interestingly, hiccoughs in the fetus can often be observed.

Week 20

The fetus is around 21 cm in length. The ears are fully functioning and can hear muffled sounds from the outside world. The fingertips have prints. The genitals can now be distinguished with an ultrasound scan.

Week 24

The fetus is around 33 cm in length. The fused eyelids now separate into upper and lower lids, enabling the baby to open and shut its eyes.

The skin is covered in fine hair (lanugo) and protected by a layer of waxy secretion (vernix). The baby makes breathing movements with its lungs.

Week 28

Your baby now weighs about 1 kg (1,000 g) or 2 lb 2oz (two pounds, two ounces) and measures about 25 cm (10 inches) from crown to rump.

The crown-to-toe length is around 37 cm. The growing body has caught up with the large head and the baby now seems more in proportion.

Week 32

The baby spends most of its time asleep. Its movements are strong and coordinated. It has probably assumed the 'head down' position by now, in preparation for birth.

Week 36

The baby is around 46 cm in length. It has probably nestled its head into its mother's pelvis, ready for birth. If it is born now, its chances for survival are excellent. Development of the lungs is rapid over the next few weeks.

Week 40

The baby is around 51 cm in length and ready to be born. It is unknown exactly what causes the onset of labour. It is most likely a combination of physical, hormonal and emotional factors between the mother and baby.

TRIMESTER WEEK BY WEEK

Pregnancy weeks are grouped into three trimesters, each one with medical milestones for both you and the baby.

First trimester

A baby grows rapidly during the first trimester (weeks 1 to 12). The fetus begins developing their brain, spinal cord, and organs. The baby's heart will also begin to beat. During the first trimester, the probability of a miscarriage is relatively high. According to the American College of Obstetricians and Gynecologists (ACOG), it's estimated that about 1 in 10 pregnancies end in miscarriage, and that about 85 percent of these occur in the first trimester.

Seek immediate help if you experience the symptoms of miscarriage.

Second trimester

During the second trimester of pregnancy (weeks 13 to 27), your healthcare provider will likely perform an anatomy scan ultrasound. This test checks the fetus's body for any developmental abnormalities. The test results can also reveal the sex of your baby, if you wish to find out before the baby is born.

You'll probably begin to feel your baby move, kick, and punch inside of your uterus.

After 23 weeks, a baby *in utero* is considered "viable." This means that it could survive living outside of your womb. Babies born this early often have serious medical issues. Your baby has a much better chance of being born healthy the longer you are able to carry the pregnancy.

Third trimester

During the third trimester (weeks 28 to 40), your weight gain will accelerate, and you may feel more tired.

Your baby can now sense light as well as open and close their eyes. Their bones are also formed.

As labor approaches, you may feel pelvic discomfort, and your feet may swell. Contractions that don't lead to labor, known as Braxton-Hicks contractions, may start to occur in the weeks before you deliver.

ANATOMIC AND PHYSIOLOGIC CHANGES OF NORMAL PREGNANCY

Changes in organs and tissues directly associated with childbearing

Ovaries

The ovaries of a nonpregnant young woman who is in good health go through cyclic changes each month. These changes centre about a follicle, or "egg sac." A new follicle develops after each menstrual period, casts off an egg (ovulation), and, after ovulation, forms a new structure (the corpus luteum).

If the egg is fertilized, it is sustained for a short time by the hormones produced by the corpus luteum. Progesterone and estrogen, secreted by the corpus luteum, are essential for the preservation of the pregnancy during its early months. If pregnancy does not occur, the egg disintegrates and the corpus luteum shrinks. As it shrinks, the stimulating effect of its hormones, progesterone and estrogen, is withdrawn from the endometrium (the lining of the uterus), and menstruation occurs. The cycle then begins again.

Pregnancy, if it occurs, maintains the corpus luteum by means of the hormones produced by the young placenta. The corpus luteum is not essential in human pregnancy after the first few weeks because of the takeover of its functions by the placenta. In fact, human pregnancies have gone on undisturbed when the corpus luteum has been removed as early as the 41st day after conception. Gradually the placenta, or afterbirth, begins to elaborate progesterone and estrogen itself. By the 70th day of pregnancy the placenta is unquestionably able to replace the corpus luteum without endangering the pregnancy during the transfer of function. At the end of pregnancy the corpus luteum has usually regressed until it is no longer a prominent feature of the ovary.

During the first few months of pregnancy the ovary that contains the functioning corpus luteum is considerably larger than the other ovary. During pregnancy, both ovaries usually are studded with fluid-filled egg sacs as a result of chorionic gonadotropin stimulation; by the end of pregnancy, most of these follicles have gradually regressed and disappeared.

The blood supply to both ovaries is increased during pregnancy. Both glands frequently reveal plaques of bright red fleshy material on their surfaces, which, if examined microscopically, demonstrate the typical cellular change of pregnancy, called a decidual reaction. In this reaction, cells develop that look like the cells in the lining of the pregnant uterus. They result from the high hormone levels that occur during pregnancy and disappear after the pregnancy terminates.

FIRST TIMERSTER PREGNANCY

Chorionic villus sampling: Answers to common questions

Chorionic villus sampling can provide valuable information about your baby's health early in pregnancy. But it's important to understand the risks — and be prepared for the results.

Prenatal testing can provide valuable information about your baby's health. But early diagnostic tests have potentially serious risks as well. If you're considering chorionic villus sampling, here's what you need to know.

What is chorionic villus sampling?: Chorionic villus sampling (CVS) is a prenatal test used to identify various genetic problems, including Down syndrome. Using a thin tube guided through your cervix or a needle inserted into your uterus, your health care provider takes a sample of chorionic villi from the placenta.

These wispy projections from the placenta — which have the same genetic makeup as your baby — transfer nutrients, oxygen and antibodies from you to your baby.

Chorionic villus sampling can provide genetic information about your baby earlier in your pregnancy than can other diagnostic tests, such as amniocentesis. The test might be offered if your baby has an increased risk of a specific chromosomal or genetic disorder. In other cases, chorionic villus sampling may be recommended if the results of a screening test in the first trimester cause concern.

Chorionic villus sampling cannot detect neural tube defects, such as spina bifida. If neural tube defects are a concern, an ultrasound or genetic amniocentesis may be recommended instead.

When is chorionic villus sampling done?: Chorionic villus sampling is usually done between the ninth and 14th weeks of pregnancy. Amniocentesis is typically done after the 15th week of pregnancy.

What happens during chorionic villus sampling?: Chorionic villus sampling can be done in the doctor's office. The procedure begins with an ultrasound to determine the position of the placenta. Then the tissue sample is taken through the cervix (transcervical) or the abdominal wall (transabdominal).

- *Transcervical CVS:* If the placenta is in a favorable position, your health care provider may take the sample through your cervix. After cleansing your vagina and cervix with an antiseptic, he or she will open your vagina with a speculum and insert a thin, hollow tube (catheter) through your cervix. When the catheter reaches the placenta, gentle suction will be used to remove a small tissue sample. You may feel cramping during the procedure.

- *Transabdominal CVS:* If the placenta isn't clearly accessible through the cervix or you have a cervical infection, such as chlamydia or herpes, your health care provider may take the sample through a needle inserted into your uterus. After cleansing your abdomen with an antiseptic, he or she will insert a long, thin needle through your abdominal wall and into your uterus. The tissue sample from the placenta will be withdrawn into a syringe, and the needle will be removed.

When are test results available?: Results may be available within two to seven days, depending on the complexity of the lab analysis.

What can chorionic villus sampling reveal?: Analysis of fetal cells can reveal whether your baby has a chromosomal abnormality, such as Down syndrome. Chorionic villus sampling can also be used to test for other genetic disorders, such as Tay-Sachs disease — but only if there is a specific reason to test for these conditions.

How accurate are the results?: With chorionic villus sampling, the chance of a false-positive — when the test is positive, but no disease exists — is less than 1 percent. But chorionic villus sampling can't identify all birth defects, including spina bifida and other neural tube defects.

What are the risks?: Chorionic villus sampling carries various risks, including:

- *Miscarriage:* Chorionic villus sampling has a one in 100 risk of miscarriage.
- *Cramping and vaginal bleeding:* You may feel cramping after the test. Vaginal bleeding also is possible, especially if the cell sample was taken through your cervix. If you develop heavy bleeding or a fever after chorionic villus sampling, contact your health care provider.
- *Rh sensitization:* Chorionic villus sampling may cause some of the baby's blood cells to enter your bloodstream. If you have Rh-negative blood and your baby has Rh-positive blood, you'll be given a drug called Rh immunoglobulin after the test to prevent you from producing antibodies against your baby's blood cells.

In the past, the risk of limb deformities was thought to be increased by chorionic villus sampling, but researchers have found no evidence to justify the initial fear. Today, chorionic villus sampling is not considered a risk factor for congenital defects of the limbs.

Chorionic villus sampling is recommended when the potential value of early diagnostic results outweighs the risk of miscarriage or other complications. Ultimately, the decision to have chorionic villus sampling is up to you. Your health care provider or genetic counselor can help you weigh all the factors in the decision.

What happens after chorionic villus sampling?: Most test results are normal, which can ease anxiety about your baby's health. Sometimes a follow-up ultrasound is recommended several days after chorionic villus sampling to verify the baby's well-being. Rarely, CVS results are unclear and amniocentesis is needed to clarify the diagnosis.

Early diagnosis of certain disorders may lead to early treatment. For example, if a female baby has congenital adrenal hyperplasia — a condition in which excessive amounts of male hormones are produced — hormone therapy can be given to the mother to prevent the baby from developing male characteristics.

If chorionic villus sampling indicates that your baby has a chromosomal problem or a genetic disorder that can't be treated, you may be faced with wrenching decisions — such as whether to continue the pregnancy. Seek support from your health care team, your loved ones and other close contacts during this difficult time.

Early pregnancy: Morning sickness, fatigue and other common symptoms

You're delighted to be pregnant, but morning sickness, heartburn, fatigue and other early-pregnancy symptoms are making your condition less than fun. Here's what to do.

Early pregnancy has its share of discomforts. Some, such as mild nausea and fatigue, are almost universal. Others, including nosebleeds and bladder infections, are less common.

Soon after you conceive, your body begins a series of major changes that enable it to sustain your baby through 37 weeks of growth and development. The glands of your endocrine system and placenta step up hormone production. Your blood volume increases and your uterus expands.

By the fourth month of pregnancy, you'll begin to feel much more like your old self, presumably because your body has adjusted somewhat to these dramatic changes. Until then, you can rest assured that first-trimester symptoms are almost always associated with normal pregnancies that have good outcomes. Morning sickness and the other ailments that occur around this time are almost always mild enough to manage on your own. Here's a rundown of the most common first-trimester symptoms.

Morning sickness

How common is it?: Up to 70 percent of expectant mothers have nausea, sometimes with vomiting, early in pregnancy.

Queasiness may be most noticeable in the morning, but it can occur at any time.

Even if you aren't nauseated, you may develop aversions to certain foods, such as coffee and meat, partly because of their odors. As long as you continue to eat a healthy diet and get all the nutrients you need, food aversions aren't a cause for concern.

What causes it?: The exact cause is unclear, but pregnancy hormones that relax the stomach may play a role.

How long does it last?: It generally improves by the 13th or 14th week of pregnancy, but some women continue to feel queasy from time to time well into the second trimester.

How can you manage it?

- Munch a few crackers before getting up in the morning.
- Eat several small meals a day so that your stomach is never empty.
- Avoid anything that causes nausea.
- Drink plenty of liquids, especially if you've been vomiting. Try crushed ice, fruit juice or frozen ice pops if water upsets your stomach.
- Try wearing a motion sickness band, which may relieve nausea by pressing on an acupressure point inside the wrist.
- Suck on hard candy.
- Try ginger, which has proved effective in combating morning sickness. Some ways to consume the spice include ginger soda or tea, gingersnaps or ginger in capsule form.

Constipation

How common is it?: Constipation affects at least half of all pregnant women.

What causes it?: An increase in the hormone progesterone, which slows the digestive process, is partly to blame. In addition, your colon absorbs more water, which tends to make stools harder and bowel movements more difficult.

How long does it last?: Infrequent, difficult-to-pass stool can be a problem any time during pregnancy, but it may be worst in the first 13 to 14 weeks.

How can you manage it?

- Try to eat on a regular schedule.
- Drink plenty of liquids — at least eight to 10 glasses a day.
- Get some exercise every day.
- Eat high-fiber fruits, vegetables and grains such as whole wheat and oatmeal.
- Try fiber supplements, such as psyllium powder, Metamucil, Konsyl, Fiberall or Citrucel. A mild laxative such as milk of magnesia is safe, but don't take any other laxative without discussing it with your doctor.

Dizziness or fainting

How common are they?: Although exact numbers aren't available, perhaps as many as one in 20 women experiences some degree of lightheadedness during pregnancy. Contrary to what's often depicted in movies, pregnant women rarely faint.

What causes them?: Pregnancy results in a dramatic dilation of the blood vessels of your body. In the first half of pregnancy, however, your blood volume may not have expanded enough to fill all of this space. The result is lower blood pressure.

Two conditions that are common during pregnancy — low blood sugar (hypoglycemia) and a low red blood cell count (anemia) — also can cause lightheadedness. The latter two causes may need medical attention.

How long do they last?: Dizziness or fainting can occur at any time during pregnancy, but may be especially noticeable early in the second trimester, when your blood vessels have dilated in response to pregnancy hormones but your blood volume hasn't yet expanded to fill them.

Fatigue

How common is it?: Almost all women report increased fatigue and need for sleep in the first trimester.

What causes it?: To carry oxygen and nutrients to the fetus, your body produces extra blood and your heart works harder and faster. These early pregnancy changes make enormous demands on your circulatory system. During this time, you're also producing higher levels of progesterone, which tends to make you sleepy. These may be factors producing the fatigue of early pregnancy.

How long does it last?: Fatigue usually subsides by the second trimester, but may return in the third trimester when carrying the extra weight of the baby may be tiring.

How can you manage it?

- *Rest:* Take naps during the day or after work. If you need to go to bed at 7 p.m. to feel rested, do so. This is a symptom that has no solution other than sleep.
- *Avoid taking on extra responsibilities:* Cut down on volunteer commitments and social events if they're wearing you out.
- *Ask for the support you need:* Get your partner or children to help out as much as possible.
- *Exercise regularly:* Moderate exercise, such as walking for 30 minutes a day, can help you feel more alert and energetic.
- *Eat foods rich in iron and protein:* Skimping on these nutrients can aggravate your fatigue. Foods rich in both iron and protein include red meat, seafood, poultry and eggs. Other good sources of iron include whole-grain or iron-fortified cereals, breads and pastas.
- *Avoid stimulants:* Avoid caffeine, which may be harmful in high doses. Any product marketed for relieving fatigue and enhancing wakefulness is unsafe in pregnancy.

Mood swings

How common are they?: Although the incidence of mood swings is unknown, some women in the first trimester and again in the weeks before delivery may experience emotional fluctuations ranging from exhilaration and joy to irritation and depression.

What causes them?: Nagging discomforts, hormonal changes and understandable anxiety about the future may all contribute to sudden shifts in your mood. You may feel better if you remind yourself that powerful emotions are normal and healthy. Simply recognizing that you're unusually moody can help you and those around you weather the storms.

How long do they last?: Mood swings may occur at any time during pregnancy. If you've typically experienced premenstrual syndrome, you may have more extreme mood swings when you're pregnant.

How can you manage them?

- Eat regular meals and snacks that include a variety of fresh fruits and vegetables and whole grains.
- Get plenty of sleep.
- Rely on your network of family and friends for support, but if you feel overwhelmed, contact your physician.
- Try relaxation techniques such as meditation, guided mental imagery and progressive muscle relaxation.

To help answer some of these questions, check out this weekly calendar of events for your baby's first three months in the womb.

Week 1: Getting ready

It may seem strange, but you're not actually pregnant the first week or two of the time allotted to your pregnancy. Yes, you read that correctly!

Conception typically occurs about two weeks after your period begins. To calculate your due date, your health care provider will count ahead 40 weeks from the start of your last period. This means your period is counted as part of your pregnancy — even though you weren't pregnant at the time.

Week 2: Fertilization

The sperm and egg unite in the fallopian tube to form a one-celled entity called a zygote. If more than one egg is released and fertilized, you may have multiple zygotes.

The zygote has 46 chromosomes — 23 from you and 23 from your partner. These chromosomes contain genetic material that will determine your baby's sex and traits such as eye colour, hair colour, height, facial features and — at least to some extent — intelligence and personality.

Soon after fertilization, the zygote will travel down one of your fallopian tubes toward the uterus. At the same time, it will begin dividing rapidly to form a cluster of cells resembling a tiny raspberry. The inner group of cells will become the embryo. The outer group of cells will become the membranes that nourish and protect it.

Week 3: Implantation

The zygote — by this time made up of about 500 cells — is now known as a blastocyst. When it reaches your uterus, the blastocyst will burrow into the uterine wall for nourishment. The placenta, which will nourish your baby throughout the pregnancy, also begins to form.

By the end of this week, you may be celebrating a positive pregnancy test.

Week 4: The embryonic period begins

The fourth week marks the beginning of the embryonic period, when the baby's brain, spinal cord, heart and other organs begin to form. Your baby is now 1/25 of an inch long.

The embryo is now made of three layers. The top layer — the ectoderm — will give rise to a groove along the midline of your baby's body. This will become the neural tube, where your baby's brain, spinal cord, spinal nerves and backbone will develop.

Your baby's heart and a primitive circulatory system will form in the middle layer of cells — the mesoderm. This layer of cells will also serve as the foundation for your baby's bones, muscles, kidneys and much of the reproductive system.

The inner layer of cells — the endoderm — will become a simple tube lined with mucous membranes. Your baby's lungs, intestines and bladder will develop here.

Week 5: Baby's heart begins to beat

At week five, your baby is 1/17 of an inch long — about the size of the tip of a pen.

This week, your baby's heart and circulatory system are taking shape. Your baby's blood vessels will complete a circuit, and his or her heart will begin to beat. Although you won't be able to hear it yet, the motion of your baby's beating heart may be detected with an ultrasound exam.

With these changes, circulation begins — making the circulatory system the first functioning organ system.

Week 6: The neural tube closes

Growth is rapid this week. Just four weeks after conception, your baby is about 1/8 of an inch long. The neural tube along your baby's back is now closed, and your baby's heart is beating with a regular rhythm.

Basic facial features will begin to appear, including an opening for the mouth and passageways that will make up the inner ear. The digestive and respiratory systems begin to form as well.

Small blocks of tissue that will form your baby's connective tissue, ribs and muscles are developing along your baby's midline. Small buds will soon grow into arms and legs.

Week 7: The umbilical cord appears

Seven weeks into your pregnancy, your baby is 1/3 of an inch long— a little bigger than the top of a pencil eraser. He or she weighs less than an aspirin tablet.

The umbilical cord — the link between your baby and the placenta— is now clearly visible. The cavities and passages needed to circulate spinal fluid in your baby's brain have formed, but your baby's skull is still transparent.

The arm bud that sprouted last week now resembles a tiny paddle. Your baby's face takes on more definition this week, as a mouth perforation, tiny nostrils and ear indentations become visible.

Week 8: Baby's fingers and toes form

Eight weeks into your pregnancy, your baby is just over 1/2 of an inch long.

Your baby will develop webbed fingers and toes this week. Wrists, elbows and ankles are clearly visible, and your baby's eyelids are beginning to form. The ears, upper lip and tip of the nose also become recognizable.

As your baby's heart becomes more fully developed, it will pump at 150 beats a minute — about twice the usual adult rate.

Week 9: Movement begins

Your baby is now nearly 1 inch long and weighs a bit less than 1/8 of an ounce. The embryonic tail at the bottom of your baby's spinal cord is shrinking, helping him or her look less like a tadpole and more like a developing person.

Your baby's head — which is nearly half the size of his or her entire body — is now tucked down onto the chest. Nipples and hair follicles begin to form. Your baby's pancreas, bile ducts, gallbladder and anus are in place. The internal reproductive organs, such as testes or ovaries, start to develop.

Your baby may begin moving this week, but you won't be able to feel for it quite a while yet.

Week 10: Neurons multiply

By now, your baby's vital organs have a solid foundation. The embryonic tail has disappeared completely, and your baby has fully separated fingers and toes. The bones of your baby's skeleton begin to form.

This week, your baby's brain will produce almost 250,000 new neurons every minute.

Your baby's eyelids are no longer transparent. The outer ears are starting to assume their final form, and tooth buds are forming as well. If your baby is a boy, his testes will start producing the male hormone testosterone.

Week 11: Baby's sex may be apparent

From now until your 20th week of pregnancy — the halfway mark— your baby will increase his or her weight 30 times and will about triple in length. To make sure your baby gets enough nutrients, the blood vessels in your placenta are growing larger and multiplying.

Your baby is now officially described as a fetus. Your baby's ears are moving up and to the side of the head this week. By the end of the week, your baby's external genitalia will develop into a recognizable penis or clitoris and labia majora.

Week 12: Baby's fingernails and toenails appear

Twelve weeks into your pregnancy, your baby is nearly 3 inches long and weighs about 4/5 of an ounce.

This week marks the arrival of fingernails and toenails. Your baby's chin and nose will become more refined as well.

Taking care of your baby: Healthy lifestyle choices — beginning even before conception — can support your baby's development. Consider these simple do's and don'ts:

Do:

- Take a prenatal vitamin or folic acid supplement.
- Maintain a healthy weight.
- Exercise regularly, with your health care provider's OK.
- Eat healthfully.
- Manage stress and any chronic health conditions.
- See your health care provider for regular prenatal checkups.
- Talk to your health care provider about any medications you're taking.

Don't:

- Smoke.
- Drink alcohol.
- Use recreational drugs.

Your baby is growing and changing every day. To give your baby the best start, take good care of yourself.

FIRST TRIMESTER PRENATAL CARE

Prenatal care is an important part of a healthy pregnancy. Here's what to expect during your initial prenatal appointments.

Prenatal care is an important part of a healthy pregnancy. Whether you choose a family physician, obstetrician or nurse-midwife, prenatal care is the key to monitoring your health — and your baby's health — throughout your pregnancy. Here's what to expect at the first few prenatal appointments.

The first visit: As soon as you think you're pregnant, schedule your first prenatal appointment. Set aside ample time for the visit. You and your health care provider have plenty to discuss! Here are the basics:

- *Medical history:* Your health care provider will ask many questions — including details about your menstrual cycle, use of contraceptives, past pregnancies, and allergies or other medical conditions. List any prescription or over-the-counter medications you're taking. Share any family history of congenital abnormalities or genetic diseases. The information you share will help your health care provider take the best care of you — and your baby.

- *Due date:* Establishing your due date early in pregnancy allows your health care provider to monitor your baby's growth as accurately as possible. To estimate your due date, your health care provider will count ahead 40 weeks from the start of your last period.

- *Physical exam:* Your health care provider will check your weight, height and blood pressure. He or she will listen to your heart and assess your overall health.

- *Pelvic exam:* Your health care provider will examine your vagina and the opening to your uterus (cervix) for any infections or abnormalities. You may need a Pap test to screen for cervical cancer. Changes in the cervix and in the size of your uterus can help confirm the stage of your pregnancy.

- *Blood tests:* Your health care provider will do blood tests to determine your blood type, including Rh factor — a specific protein on the surface of red blood cells. Blood tests also can reveal whether you've been exposed to syphilis, measles, mumps, rubella or hepatitis B. You may be offered a test for HIV, the virus that causes AIDS. Tests for chickenpox and toxoplasmosis immunity may be done as well.

- *Urine tests:* Analysis of your urine can reveal a bladder or kidney infection. The presence of too much sugar or protein in your urine may suggest diabetes or kidney disease.
- *Lifestyle issues:* Healthy lifestyle choices can help give your baby the best start. Your health care provider will talk to you about nutrition, prenatal vitamins, exercise and other lifestyle issues. You'll also discuss your work environment. If you smoke, your health care provider will offer suggestions to help you quit.
- *Prenatal tests:* Prenatal tests can give you valuable information about your baby's health. Your health care provider may recommend ultrasound, blood tests or other screening tests to detect fetal abnormalities.

Other first-trimester visits: Subsequent prenatal visits — often scheduled every four to six weeks during the first trimester — will probably be shorter than the first. Your health care provider will check your weight and blood pressure, and you'll discuss your signs and symptoms. You probably won't need another pelvic exam until later in your pregnancy. Near the end of the first trimester, you may be able to hear your baby's heartbeat with a small device that bounces sound waves off your baby's heart.

Remember, your health care provider is there to support you throughout your pregnancy. Your prenatal appointments are an ideal time to discuss any questions or concerns — including things that may be uncomfortable or embarrassing. Also find out how to reach your health care provider between appointments. Knowing help is available when you need it can offer precious peace of mind.

Pregnancy: Symptoms and emotions in the first trimester

Early pregnancy brings many symptoms, but evidence of your pregnancy remains invisible for now.

The first few months of pregnancy are marked by an invisible — yet amazing — transformation. Knowing what to expect can help you face the months ahead with confidence.

Your body: Within two weeks of conception, hormones trigger your body to begin nourishing the baby — even before tests and a physical exam can confirm the pregnancy. Here are some common physical changes you may notice early on.

- *Tender breasts:* Increased hormone production may make your breasts unusually sensitive. Your breasts will probably feel fuller and heavier. Wearing a more supportive bra may help.

- *Bouts of nausea:* Many women have queasiness, nausea or vomiting in early pregnancy — probably due to normal hormonal changes. Nausea tends to be worse in the morning, but it can last all day.

Eat small, frequent meals throughout the day to help relieve this pregnancy symptom. Suck on hard candy. Try ginger ale or ginger tea. Avoid foods or smells that make your nausea worse.

- *Unusual fatigue:* You may feel tired as your body produces more blood and prepares to support the pregnancy. Your heart will pump faster and harder, and your pulse will quicken. Intense, changeable emotions also may take a toll on your energy level.

If you're fatigued, rest as much as you can. Make sure you're getting enough iron and protein. Include physical activity in your daily routine, such as a brisk walk.

- *Dizziness:* Normal circulatory changes in early pregnancy may leave you feeling a little dizzy. Stress, fatigue and hunger also may play a role.

To prevent mild, occasional dizziness, avoid prolonged standing. Rise slowly after lying or sitting down. Keep blood sugar from falling with occasional snacks, such as dried fruit or low-fat yogurt. If you start to feel dizzy while you're driving, pull over. If you're standing when dizziness hits, sit or lie down.

Contact your health care provider if the dizziness is severe and occurs with abdominal pain or vaginal bleeding. Rarely, this may indicate an ectopic pregnancy, in which the fertilized egg implants itself outside the uterus.

- *Increased urination:* You may need to urinate more often as your uterus presses on your bladder during the first few months of pregnancy. The same pressure may cause you to leak urine when sneezing, coughing or laughing.

To help prevent urinary tract infections, urinate whenever you feel the need to. If you're losing sleep due to middle-of-the-night bathroom trips, drink less fluid in the evening. If you're worried about leaking urine, panty liners may help you feel more secure.

Your emotions: Pregnancy may leave you feeling delighted, anxious, exhilarated and exhausted — sometimes all at once. Even if you're thrilled about being pregnant, a new baby adds emotional stress to your life.

It's natural to worry about your baby's health, your adjustment to motherhood and the increased financial demands of raising a child. You may wonder how the baby will affect your relationship with your partner or what type of parents you'll be. If you work outside the home, you may worry about your productivity on the job and how to balance the competing demands of family and career.

You may also experience misgivings and bouts of weepiness or mood swings. To cope with these emotions, remind yourself that what you're feeling is normal. Take good care of yourself, and look to your partner and family for understanding and encouragement. If the mood changes become severe or intense, consult your health care provider for additional support.

Your relationship with your partner: Becoming a mother takes time away from other roles and relationships. You may lose some of your psychological identity as a partner and lover — but good communication can help you keep the intimacy alive.

- *Be honest:* Let your partner know that you need his presence, support and tenderness — sometimes without sexual overtones. Identify the stress points in your relationship before they become problematic.
- *Be patient:* Occasional misunderstandings and conflicts

are inevitable. Consider both sides. If your partner dives into his work, for example, you may feel hurt and rejected because it appears as though he's withdrawing from your relationship. Your partner, on the other hand, may simply be trying to provide more security for your family.

- *Be supportive:* Encourage your partner to identify his doubts and worries and be honest about what he's feeling — both the good and the bad. Do the same yourself. Discussing your feelings honestly and openly will strengthen your relationship and help you begin preparing a home for your baby.

Appointments with your health care provider: Whether you choose a family physician, obstetrician or nurse-midwife, your health care provider will treat, educate and reassure you throughout your pregnancy. He or she is there to help you celebrate the miracle of birth.

Your first visit will focus mainly on assessing your overall health, identifying any risk factors and determining your baby's gestational age. Your health care provider will ask lots of questions about your health history. Be honest. The answers you provide will help you and your baby receive the best care.

After the first visit, you may be asked to schedule checkups every four to six weeks until the last month of your pregnancy, when you may need checkups every week or two. During these appointments, raise any concerns or fears you may have about pregnancy, childbirth or life with a newborn. No question is silly or unimportant — and the answers can help you take the best care of yourself and your baby.

SECOND TIMESTER PREGNANCY

Amniocentesis: Answers to common questions

Amniocentesis can provide valuable information about your baby's health. But it's important to understand the risks — and be prepared for the results.

Prenatal testing can provide valuable information about your baby's health. But the decision to pursue invasive diagnostic tests is serious. If you're considering amniocentesis, here's what you need to know.

What is amniocentesis?: Amniocentesis is a prenatal test used to identify various genetic problems or test a baby's lung maturity. Using a thin needle inserted into your uterus, your health care provider withdraws a sample of the amniotic fluid that surrounds and protects the baby. This fluid contains fetal cells and various chemicals produced by the baby.

With genetic amniocentesis, the chromosomes and genes in these cells or the chemicals in the amniotic fluid can be tested for certain abnormalities, such as Down syndrome and spina bifida. With maturity amniocentesis, the amniotic fluid is tested to determine whether a baby's lungs are mature enough for birth.

Who might need amniocentesis?: Genetic amniocentesis is typically offered to women age 35 or older, whose babies have an increased risk of chromosomal abnormalities. Other reasons to consider genetic amniocentesis include:

- A chromosomal abnormality or neural tube defect in a previous pregnancy
- Abnormal results from a prenatal screening test, such as first trimester screening or the quad marker screen
- A family history of central nervous system defects, Down syndrome or other genetic disorders

Maturity amniocentesis — to determine whether the baby's lungs are ready for birth — is only needed if early delivery would be best for the mother.

When is amniocentesis done?: Genetic amniocentesis is usually done after the 15th week of pregnancy. At this point, the two layers of fetal membranes have fused enough to safely withdraw a sample of amniotic fluid for evaluation. Maturity amniocentesis is most common after the 36th week of pregnancy.

What happens during amniocentesis?: Amniocentesis can be done in the doctor's office. Your health care provider will use ultrasound to determine the baby's exact location in your uterus. Then your abdomen will be cleaned with an antiseptic. Guided by ultrasound, your health care provider will insert a thin, hollow needle through your abdominal wall and into your uterus. About 2 to 4 teaspoons of amniotic fluid will be withdrawn into a syringe, and the needle will be removed.

You'll notice a stinging sensation when the needle enters your skin. Many women feel mild cramps as the needle passes through the uterus. The baby quickly replaces the small amount of fluid that's removed.

When are test results available?: The sample of amniotic fluid is analyzed in a lab. For genetic analysis, some results may be available within a few days. Traditional chromosomal assessment takes up to 14 days — long enough for the fetal cells to multiply until there are enough to be tested. Results of maturity amniocentesis are available within hours.

What can amniocentesis reveal?: Genetic amniocentesis can identify chromosomal abnormalities and certain genetic problems, including Down syndrome and spina bifida. Many other conditions — including cystic fibrosis, hemophilia and sickle cell disease — can be diagnosed using amniocentesis as well, but only if there is a specific reason to test for these conditions.

Less often, amniocentesis is used to diagnose uterine infections or Rh incompatibility — an uncommon condition in which a mother's immune system produces antibodies against a specific protein on the surface of the baby's blood cells.

By analyzing the types of compounds produced in the baby's lungs, maturity amniocentesis can determine if the baby is ready to breathe air.

Fetal development

As your pregnancy progresses, your baby will begin to seem more real. You may be amazed by how much your baby changes from week to week. As your pregnancy progresses, your baby will begin to seem more real. You may hear the heartbeat at your prenatal appointments, and your growing abdomen may force your favorite jeans to the back of the closet.

While you're adjusting to the changes in your body, your baby is quickly maturing. Two months ago, your baby was simply a cluster of cells. Now, he or she has functioning organs, nerves and muscles. You may be amazed by how much your baby changes from week to week.

Week 13: Baby flexes and kicks

You can't feel it yet, but your baby can move in a jerky fashion — flexing the arms and kicking the legs. This week, your baby might even be able to put a thumb in his or her mouth.

Your baby's eyelids are fused together to protect his or her developing eyes. Tissue that will become bone is developing around your baby's head and within the arms and legs. Tiny ribs may soon appear.

Week 14: Hormones gear up

The effect of hormones becomes apparent this week. For boys, the prostate gland is developing. For girls, the ovaries move from the abdomen into the pelvis.

Meconium — which will become your baby's first bowel movement after birth — is made in your baby's intestinal tract. By the end of the week, the roof of your baby's mouth will be completely formed.

Week 15: Skin begins to form

Your baby's skin starts out nearly transparent. Eyebrows and scalp hair may make an appearance. For babies destined to have dark hair, the hair follicles will begin producing pigment.

The bone and marrow that make up your baby's skeletal system are continuing to develop this week. Your baby's eyes and ears now have a baby-like appearance, and the ears have almost reached their final position.

Week 16: Facial expressions are possible

Sixteen weeks into your pregnancy, your baby is between 4 and 5 inches long and weighs a bit less than 3 ounces. He or she can now make a fist.

Your baby's eyes are becoming sensitive to light. More developed facial muscles may lead to various expressions, such as squinting and frowning. Your baby may have frequent bouts of hiccups as well. For girls, millions of eggs are forming in the ovaries.

Week 17: Fat accumulates

Fat stores begin to develop under your baby's skin this week. The fat will provide energy and help keep your baby warm after birth.

Week 18: Baby begins to hear

As the nerve endings from your baby's brain "hook up" to the ears, your baby may hear your heart beating, your stomach rumbling or blood moving through the umbilical cord. He or she may even be startled by loud noises. Your baby can swallow this week, too.

Week 19: Lanugo covers baby's skin

Your baby's delicate skin is now protected with a pasty white coating called vernix. Under the vernix, a fine, down-like hair called lanugo covers your baby's body. Your baby's kidneys are already producing urine. The urine is excreted into the amniotic sac, which surrounds and protects your baby.

As your baby's hearing continues to improve, he or she may pick up your voice in conversations — although it's probably hard to hear clearly through the amniotic fluid and protective paste covering your baby's ears.

Thanks to the millions of motor neurons developing in the brain, your baby can make reflexive muscle movements. If you haven't felt movement yet, you will soon.

Week 20: The halfway point

Halfway into your pregnancy, your baby is about 6 inches long and weighs about 9 ounces — a little over half a pound. You've probably begun to feel your baby's movements. Under the protection of the vernix, your baby's skin is thickening and developing layers. Your baby now has thin eyebrows, hair on the scalp and well-developed limbs.

Week 21: Nourishment evolves

Although the placenta provides nearly all of your baby's nourishment, your baby will begin to absorb small amounts of sugar from swallowed amniotic fluid. This week, your baby's bone marrow starts making blood cells — a job done by the liver and spleen until this point.

Week 22: Taste buds develop

This week, your baby weighs in at about 1 pound.

Taste buds are starting to form on your baby's tongue, and your baby's brain and nerve endings can process the sensation of touch. Your baby may experiment by feeling his or her face or anything else within reach.

For boys, the testes begin to descend from the abdomen this week. For girls, the uterus and ovaries are in place — complete with a lifetime supply of eggs.

Week 23: Lungs prepare for life outside the womb

Your baby's lungs are beginning to produce surfactant, the substance that allows the air sacs in the lungs to inflate — and keeps them from collapsing and sticking together when they deflate. "Practice" breathing moves amniotic fluid in and out of your baby's lungs.

Your baby will begin to look more like a newborn as the skin becomes less transparent and fat production kicks into high gear.

With intensive medical care, some babies born at 23 weeks can survive. There are serious risks, however, such as bleeding in the brain and impaired vision. Advances in fetal medicine are steadily improving the odds for the tiniest preemies.

Week 24: Sense of balance develops

By now, your baby weighs about 1 1/2 pounds. Footprints and fingerprints are forming.

Thanks to a fully developed inner ear, which controls balance, your baby may have a sense of whether he or she is upside-down or right side up in the womb. You may notice a regular sleeping and waking cycle. Babies born at 24 weeks have more than a 50 percent chance of survival. The odds get better with every passing week. Still, complications are frequent and serious.

Week 25: Exploration continues

Your baby's hands are now fully developed, although the nerve connections to the hands have a long way to go. Exploring the structures inside your uterus may become baby's prime entertainment.

Week 26: Eyes remain closed

Your baby weighs between 1 1/2 and 2 pounds. The eyebrows and eyelashes are well formed, and the hair on your baby's head is longer and more plentiful. Although your baby's eyes are fully developed, they may not open for another two weeks.

Week 27: Second trimester ends

This week marks the end of the second trimester. Your baby's lungs, liver and immune system are continuing to mature — and he or she has been growing like a weed. At 27 weeks, your baby's length will have tripled or even quadrupled from the 12-week mark.

If your baby is born this week, the chance of survival is at least 85 percent. However, serious complications are still possible.

Taking care of your baby: Healthy lifestyle choices throughout pregnancy will support your baby's development. Consider these simple do's and don'ts:

Do:
- Take a prenatal vitamin.
- Maintain a healthy weight.
- Exercise regularly, with your health care provider's OK.
- Eat healthfully.
- Manage stress and any chronic health conditions.
- See your health care provider for regular prenatal checkups.

Don't:
- Smoke.

- Drink alcohol.
- Take medication without your health care provider's OK.

Your baby is growing and changing every day — and so are you. Marvel at the changes as you anticipate what's to come.

PREGNANCY: SYMPTOMS AND EMOTIONS IN THE SECOND TRIMESTER

Now's the time to enjoy your pregnancy. You may be feeling better than ever.

The second trimester of pregnancy often brings a renewed sense of well-being. The worst of the nausea has usually passed, and your baby isn't big enough to crowd your abdominal organs and make you uncomfortable. Yet dramatic physical and emotional changes are on the horizon. Here's what to expect.

Your body: As your pregnancy progresses, you may notice physical changes from head to toe.

- *Larger breasts:* Stimulated by estrogen and progesterone, the milk-producing glands inside your breasts get larger. A small amount of fat may also accumulate in your breasts. The result may be as much as 1 pound of extra breast tissue or up to two additional cup sizes.
- *Growing belly:* As your uterus becomes heavier and expands to make room for the baby, your abdomen expands right along with it. Expect to gain up to 4 pounds a month until the end of your pregnancy.
- *Braxton Hicks contractions:* Your uterus may start flexing to build strength for the big job ahead. You may feel these warm-ups, called Braxton Hicks contractions, in your lower abdomen and groin. They're painless and come and go unpredictably. Contact your health care provider if the contractions become painful or regular. This may be a sign of preterm labour.
- *Skin changes:* As blood circulation increases, you may enjoy the healthy glow associated with pregnancy. Certain areas of your skin may become darker as well, such as the skin around your nipples, parts of your face and the line that runs from your navel to your pubic bone.

- *Nasal and gum problems:* As pregnancy expands your circulation, more blood flows through your body's mucous membranes, causing the lining of your nose and airway to swell. This can restrict airflow and cause snoring, congestion and nosebleeds. Increased blood circulation can soften your gums as well, which may cause minor bleeding when you brush or floss your teeth.

- *Dizziness:* Your blood vessels dilate in response to pregnancy hormones. Until your blood volume expands to fill them, you may experience occasional dizziness. Lower blood pressure due to your rapidly expanding circulatory system also may play a role. Avoid prolonged standing, and rise slowly after lying or sitting down.

- *Leg cramps:* During the second trimester of pregnancy, pressure from your uterus on the veins returning blood from your legs may cause leg cramps, especially at night. Stretch the affected muscle or walk your way through the cramps.

- *Heartburn and constipation:* During pregnancy, the movements that push swallowed food from your esophagus into your stomach are slower. Your stomach also takes longer to empty. This slowdown gives nutrients more time to be absorbed into your bloodstream and reach your baby. Unfortunately, it may also lead to heartburn and constipation.

- *Shortness of breath:* Your lungs are processing up to 40 percent more air than they did before your pregnancy. This allows your blood to carry large quantities of oxygen to your placenta and the baby — and may leave you breathing slightly faster and feeling short of breath.

- *Vaginal discharge:* You may notice a thin, white vaginal discharge. This acidic discharge is thought to help suppress the growth of potentially harmful bacteria. Contact your health care provider if the discharge becomes strong-smelling, green or yellowish or it's accompanied by redness, itching or irritation. This may indicate a vaginal infection.

- *Bladder and kidney infections:* Hormonal changes slow

the flow of urine, and your expanding uterus also may get in the way — both factors that increase the risk of bladder and kidney infections. Contact your health care provider if you need to urinate more often than usual, you notice a burning sensation when you urinate, or you have a fever, abdominal pain or backache. Left untreated, these infections may increase the risk of preterm labour.

Your emotions: Pregnancy is a psychological journey as well as a biological one. During the second trimester, you may feel less moody and more up to the challenge of preparing a home for your baby. Strike while the iron is hot! Check into childbirth classes. Find a health care provider for your baby. Read about breast-feeding. If you plan to work outside the home after the baby is born, get familiar with your company's maternity leave policy and investigate child care options.

As your pregnancy progresses, changes in your body's shape and function may affect your emotions. Some women feel a heightened sexuality during pregnancy. Others feel unattractive — especially as their bellies grow. If you're struggling with your body image, share your concerns with your partner. Express love and affection in ways that help you feel most comfortable.

While anticipation mounts, worries about labour, delivery or impending motherhood may preoccupy you. Remember that you can't plan or control everything about your pregnancy. Instead, focus on making healthy lifestyle choices that will give your baby the best start.

Appointments with your health care provider: During the second trimester, your prenatal appointments will focus on your baby's growth, confirming your due date and detecting any problems with your health.

Your health care provider will begin by checking your weight and blood pressure. He or she may measure the size of your uterus by checking the fundal height — the distance from the top of the uterus (called the fundus) to your pubic bone. Pelvic exams are often unnecessary during the second trimester, unless something unusual needs to be explored.

At this stage, the highlight of your prenatal visits may be listening to your baby's heartbeat with a special device called a Doppler. Your doctor may suggest an ultrasound or other screening tests this trimester.

Be sure to mention any signs or symptoms that concern you, even if they seem silly or unimportant. Talking to your health care provider is likely to put your mind at ease.

SECOND TRIMESTER PRENATAL CARE

As your pregnancy progresses, you'll continue to visit your health care provider regularly. Here's what to expect during prenatal appointments in the second trimester.

As your pregnancy progresses, prenatal care remains important. You'll continue to visit your health care provider regularly — probably once a month throughout the second trimester. Here's what to expect at your prenatal appointments.

Covering the basics: Your health care provider will check your blood pressure and weight at every visit. Mention any signs or symptoms you've been experiencing. Then it's time for your baby to take center stage. Your health care provider may:

- *Track your baby's growth:* By measuring your abdomen from the top of your uterus to your pubic bone, your health care provider can gauge your baby's growth. This measurement in centimeters often equals the number of weeks of pregnancy.
- *Listen to your baby's heartbeat:* You'll hear your baby's heartbeat, too, thanks to a special device called a Doppler.
- *Assess fetal movement:* Tell your health care provider when you begin noticing flutters or kicks — often by 20 weeks.

Expect routine lab tests: Your health care provider may want to test a urine sample for sugar and protein. You may need blood tests to check for low iron levels or gestational diabetes, a temporary form of diabetes that can develop during pregnancy. If you have Rh negative blood, you may be tested for Rh antibodies. These antibodies may be harmful if your baby has Rh positive blood.

Consider prenatal testing: During the second trimester, you may be offered various prenatal screenings or tests.

- *Blood tests:* Blood tests may be done to screen for developmental or chromosomal disorders, such as spina bifida or Down syndrome.
- *Ultrasound:* An ultrasound can help your health care provider evaluate your baby's growth and development. It also gives you an exciting glimpse of your baby.
- *Diagnostic tests:* If the results of a blood test or ultrasound are worrisome, your health care provider may recommend a more invasive diagnostic test, such as amniocentesis.

Keep your health care provider informed: The second trimester often brings a renewed sense of well-being. But there's a lot happening. Tell your health care provider what's on your mind, even if it seems silly or unimportant. Nothing is too trivial when it comes to your health — or your baby's health.

THIRD TIMESTER PREGNANCY

Back pain during pregnancy

You can develop back pain at any stage of pregnancy. The causes vary, but a few simple steps will usually bring relief.

As your pregnancy advances and your uterus enlarges, you're likely to feel some discomfort. Back pain is a common complaint.

But you don't have to grin and accept back pain as a normal part of your pregnancy. You can take steps to stop the soreness. It's a good idea to learn these techniques now, because you'll probably need them again later when your back is bearing the strain of constantly lifting your 7- to 10-pound baby or your 20-pound toddler.

What causes back pain in pregnancy?: At least 50 percent of women experience back pain during pregnancy. Pregnant women are prone to backaches and back pain for a number of reasons:

- *Extra weight:* The weight you gain during pregnancy is good for your baby, but it can be bad for your back.
- *Change in center of gravity:* As your uterus grows, your

center of gravity shifts forward. Gradually — and perhaps without notice — you begin to adjust your posture and the way you move. These compensations can lead to backaches and back pain.

- *Your hormones:* During pregnancy, the hormone relaxin causes the ligaments between your pelvic bones to soften and your joints to loosen in preparation for your baby's passage through your pelvis during birth. As the structures that support your pelvic organs become more pliant, you may feel considerable discomfort on either side of your lower back, often with walking, especially up and down stairs.

Back pain can occur at any time during pregnancy. For many women, it interferes with daily activities and the ability to get a good night's sleep.

What can you do?: These self-care strategies can put your back on track:

- *Pay attention to your posture:* The healthy posture that you learned before you were pregnant still applies in early pregnancy, before your uterus is above your bellybutton. Tuck your buttocks under, pull your shoulders back and downward, and stand straight and tall.

Later in pregnancy, as your uterus enlarges, you naturally pull your shoulders back farther to offset the weight of your uterus pulling you forward. This can actually cause back strain. Talk to your doctor about adjusting your posture to accommodate your growing belly.

- *Make adjustments when sitting or standing:* Sit with your feet slightly elevated, and don't cross your legs. Change position often, and avoid standing for long periods of time. If you must stand for a while, rest one foot on a low step stool.

- *Strategically place your pillows:* Sleep on your side, with one or both knees bent. Place a pillow between your knees and another one under your abdomen. You may also find relief by placing a specially shaped total body pillow under your abdomen.

- *Avoid lifting heavy objects or children:* When lifting a smaller object, don't bend over at the waist. Instead, squat down, bend your knees and lift with your legs rather than your back. Try to avoid sudden reaching movements or stretching your arms high over your head.
- *Get the right gear:* Wear supportive, low-heeled shoes and maternity pants with a low, supportive waistband. Or consider using a maternity support belt.
- *Try heat, cold or massage:* Apply heat to your back. Try warm bath soaks, warm wet towels, a hot water bottle or a heating pad. Some women find relief by alternating ice packs with heat. A back massage also may help.
- *Stay fit:* As long as your health care provider approves, an exercise programme can keep your back strong and may actually relieve back pain. Some women enjoy swimming, and doctors highly recommend it — the body's buoyancy in the water offers relief from the extra weight of pregnancy. You also might like walking or taking a prenatal exercise or yoga class. On your own, you can try an exercise called a pelvic tilt or cat stretch: Kneel on your hands and knees with your head in line with your back. Pull in your abdomen, arching your spine upward. Hold the position for several seconds, then relax your abdomen and back. Repeat three to five times, working gradually up to 10.

If these self-care steps aren't working or your back pain is severe, talk to your health care provider. He or she may suggest a variety of approaches, such as special stretching exercises, that can alleviate pain without causing concern for your unborn baby.

Pain in your back may be a sign of a more serious problem if it's severe and unrelenting or if it's accompanied by other signs and symptoms. A low, dull backache may be a sign of labour or preterm labour. So, it's best not to ignore your aching back.

Childbirth education: Get ready for labour and delivery

Do you know what to expect during labour and delivery? Whether you're a first-time mom or a delivery room veteran, here's why you should take a class. By now, you've probably surrounded yourself with articles on childbirth and heard countless labour stories from friends and loved ones. But do you really know what to expect during labour and delivery? A childbirth education class can make all the difference.

Why should I take a childbirth education class?: Whether you're a first-time mom or a delivery room veteran, a childbirth education class can help you prepare to meet the challenges of labour and delivery. Consider the opportunities:

- *Learn things you never knew about labour, delivery and postpartum care:* You'll find out what happens to your body as your baby makes his or her way into the world — from just how messy delivery can be to why you may need to leave your contact lenses at home.

- *Address your fears:* What if I don't make it to the hospital in time? What if I lose control during labour? During class, you'll have the chance to talk about your fears with other couples who probably share the same concerns. The instructor can dispel myths and help put your mind at ease.

- *Connect with your partner or labour coach:* A class offers your partner or labour coach the chance to learn about childbirth, too— as well as how to support you during labour.

- *Discuss options for handling pain:* You'll practice various methods for coping with contractions, such as breathing, relaxation and visualization. Most classes also cover the pros and cons of common medications, such as narcotic analgesics and epidural blocks.

- *Get the basics on Caesarean delivery:* You'll learn why a C-section may be needed — and what to expect if it happens to you.

- *Check out the facility:* You'll probably tour the facility and see various devices that may be used during labour or delivery, such as a fetal monitor. A preview leaves fewer surprises for the big day.

- *Brush up on newborn care:* In addition to labour and delivery, you'll get a primer on newborns. Common topics include breast-feeding, diapering, bathing and comforting.
- *Gain a sense of control:* Knowledge is power. You'll feel less vulnerable during labour and delivery if you understand what's happening.

Are there different types of childbirth education classes?: Yes. Some classes cover specific types of births, such as Caesarean birth, vaginal birth after Caesarean section (VBAC) and multiple births. Refresher courses are available for people who simply want to review the basics. Other classes focus on specific methods of childbirth. For example:

- *Lamaze:* The goal of Lamaze is to increase confidence in your ability to give birth. Lamaze classes help you learn how to respond to pain in ways that both facilitate labour and promote comfort — including focused breathing, movement and massage.
- *Bradley:* This method considers birth a natural process. You're encouraged to trust your body, focusing on diet and exercise throughout pregnancy. You're taught to manage labour through relaxation, deep breathing and the support of a husband or partner.

You may also find classes on other approaches to childbirth, including hypnotherapy, water birth — even using art to work through birthing issues.

What's the best way to find a class?: Childbirth preparation classes are offered at most hospitals and birthing centers. Some classes are available online or in video format. Ask your health care provider about available classes. A local childbirth association may offer suggestions as well. Try the International Childbirth Education Association or similar groups.

When should I take the class?: Childbirth education classes are often recommended near the sixth or seventh month of pregnancy — but anytime before you go into labour would be helpful. Classes are often offered as one- to two-hour sessions over the course of several months or as full-day weekend sessions. The earlier you register, the more options and flexibility you'll have regarding class dates and times.

How much will it cost?; That depends. Short courses may be offered for a nominal fee. More intense courses may cost $100 or more. Some insurance plans offer reduced registration fees or reimbursement plans for childbirth courses. Fees at some facilities may be based on your ability to pay.

What is my health care provider's role?: Your health care provider is there to help you have a positive birth experience. With his or her input, use what you learn in your childbirth class to create a birth plan. No one can predict how the birth will go, but together you can design a birth plan that meets your expectations for labour, delivery and postpartum care— and promotes the best care for you and your baby.

FETAL DEVELOPMENT

Your baby continues to grow and change every week as your due date approaches. Here's a look at what's going on.

The countdown is on! By now, you may be tired of being pregnant— and eager to meet your baby face-to-face. But your uterus is still a busy place. Check out how much your baby continues to grow and develop as your due date approaches.

Week 28: Baby's eyes open

Your baby is about 15 inches long and weighs about 2 to 3 pounds.

Your baby's eyes are beginning to open and close. The colour has been established, but the story's not over yet. Eye colour may change within the first six months of life — especially if your baby's eyes are blue or gray-blue at birth.

Your baby is now sleeping for about 20 to 30 minutes at a time. Fetal movement will be most obvious when you're sitting or lying down.

Week 29: Movement is more forceful

Your baby's bones are fully developed, but they're still soft and pliable. This week, your baby begins storing iron, calcium and phosphorus. As your baby continues to grow, his or her movements will become more frequent and vigorous. Some of your baby's jabs and punches may even take your breath away.

Week 30: Baby packs on pounds

Your baby weighs about 3 pounds — but not for long. He or she will gain about 1/2 pound a week until week 37. Your baby may practice breathing by moving his or her diaphragm in a repeating rhythm. If your baby gets the hiccups, you may feel slight twitches or spasms in your uterus.

Week 31: Reproductive development continues

If your baby is a boy, his testicles are moving from their location near the kidneys through the groin on their way into the scrotum. If your baby is a girl, her clitoris is now relatively prominent.

Your baby's lungs are more developed, but they're not fully mature. If your baby is born this week, he or she will probably need a ventilator to breathe. Complications such as bleeding in the brain are less likely than they were even a few weeks ago.

Week 32: Downy hair falls off

Your baby is between 15 and 17 inches long and weighs about 4 to 4 1/2 pounds. Nearly all babies born at this age survive the challenges of premature birth.

The layer of soft, downy hair that has covered your baby's skin for the past few months — known as lanugo — starts to fall off this week.

As space in your uterus becomes more cramped, your baby's kicks and other movements may seem less forceful. You may want to check on your baby's movements from time to time — especially if you think you've noticed decreased activity. If you count fewer than 10 movements in two hours, contact your health care provider.

Week 33: Baby detects light

Your baby's pupils now constrict, dilate and detect light. Your baby continues to gain about 1/2 pound a week, and his or her lungs are more completely developed. Babies born this week need extra attention, but almost all will be healthy.

Week 34: Protective coating gets thicker

The pasty white coating that protects your baby's skin — called vernix — gets thicker this week. When your baby is born, you may see traces of vernix firsthand, especially under the arms, behind the ears and in the groin area. The soft, downy hair that covered your baby under the vernix for the past few months is now almost completely gone.

Week 35: Rapid growth continues

Your baby continues to pack on the pounds and store fat all over his or her body. The crowded conditions inside your uterus may make it harder for your baby to give you a punch, but you'll probably feel lots of stretches, rolls and wiggles.

Week 36: Baby can suck

Your baby is between 16 and 19 inches long and weighs about 6 to 6 1/2 pounds. Recent fat deposits have rounded out your baby's face, and your baby's powerful sucking muscles are ready for action. To prepare for birth, your baby may descend into the head down position.

Week 37: Baby is full-term

By the end of this week, your baby will be considered full-term. As fat continues to accumulate, your baby's body will slowly become rounder.

Week 38: Organ function continues to improve

Your baby weighs nearly 7 pounds. His or her brain and nervous system are working better every day. This developmental process will continue through childhood and adolescence.

Week 39: Placenta provides antibodies

Your baby has enough fat under the skin to hold his or her body temperature as long as there's a little help from you. The placenta continues to supply your baby with antibodies that will help fight infection the first six months after birth. If you breast-feed your baby, your milk will provide additional antibodies.

Week 40: Your due date arrives

Your baby may be 19 to 21 inches long and weigh 7 to 8 pounds.

Don't be alarmed if your due date comes and goes without incident. It's just as normal to deliver a baby a week late — or a week early — than it is to deliver right on time. In fact, only an estimated 5 percent of women deliver on their due dates.

Taking care of your baby: Although your pregnancy is nearly over, healthy lifestyle choices remain important. Remember these simple do's and don'ts:

Do:

- Take a prenatal vitamin.
- Maintain a healthy weight.
- Exercise regularly, with your health care provider's OK.
- Eat healthfully.
- Manage stress and any chronic health conditions.
- See your health care provider for regular prenatal checkups — probably once a week for the last month of pregnancy.

Don't:

- Smoke.
- Drink alcohol.
- Take medication without your health care provider's OK.

Enjoy the final days of your pregnancy. This is it! The next chapter in your life is about to begin.

Group B strep: How to protect your baby

Group B strep is common and usually harmless in adults, but it causes serious illness and death in newborns. Protect your baby with third-trimester testing.

Try as you might, it's impossible to protect your new baby from every cold and virus going around. But you can usually prevent one of the most common causes of serious illness and death in newborns — group B streptococcus (GBS).

This bacterium — which is in the same family as the germ that causes strep throat — is common and usually harmless in adults. However, pregnant women who harbour GBS may pass it to their babies during labour and delivery. If you're pregnant, you can detect this problem and make plans to stop it by taking a GBS test during your third trimester.

Harmless in adults, dangerous for babies: Many adults — including 25 percent of pregnant women in the United States — have group B strep in their bodies, usually in the bowel, bladder, vagina, rectum or throat. In adults with serious medical conditions, such as liver failure or cancer, GBS can cause dangerous infections. But most adults are just carriers of the bacterium, which means they have no symptoms and don't feel sick. In fact, GBS in adults usually isn't treated because it usually isn't harmful.

Pregnant women with GBS are the exception, because they can pass the bacteria to their babies during vaginal delivery. Doctors and researchers think this happens when a baby passes through the birth canal and comes into contact with — or swallows — fluids containing GBS bacteria.

Only a very small number of babies born to women carrying group B strep become infected, but these babies can become critically ill. Premature babies are much more likely to be affected by GBS disease, but it can rarely affect full-term babies. There are two forms of GBS disease in infants — early-onset and late-onset.

Early-onset GBS disease: This is the more common and serious form of GBS infection in infants. In this form of the infection, a baby typically becomes sick within hours after birth. The infection usually starts with fever, difficulty feeding and lethargy. But it can lead to:

- *Pneumonia,* an infection and inflammation of the lungs
- *Sepsis,* a potentially life-threatening condition that occurs when infection spreads throughout the bloodstream
- *Meningitis,* an infection and inflammation of the membranes and fluid surrounding the brain and spinal cord

Late-onset GBS disease: Late-onset GBS disease develops within a week to a few months after birth. About half the cases of late-onset disease are acquired from the mother. The exact source of the other cases is unknown. Problems associated with late-onset GBS disease can be similar to early-onset GBS. However, the impact is usually somewhat less severe.

If you suspect that your baby has either form of GBS disease or one of its complications, see your doctor right away. A blood test and culture can confirm the problem, so your baby can start antibiotic treatment. Despite antibiotics, both early- and late-onset GBS can be fatal. And babies who survive can have long-term neurological damage, including seizures and hearing loss, particularly following meningitis.

How to know if you have GBS?: Most cases of GBS disease in infants can be prevented by screening and appropriate treatment during labour. The Centers for Disease Control and Prevention currently recommends that that all pregnant women undergo GBS screening between 35 and 37 weeks of gestation during each pregnancy.

GBS screening involves a simple swab of the vagina and the rectum that can be tested for the bacterium in a laboratory. A positive test indicates that you're a carrier of GBS, but it doesn't necessarily mean that your baby will become ill. Antibiotics given intravenously during labour can kill some of the strep bacteria that are dangerous to your baby during birth. Antibiotics aren't guaranteed to prevent GBS, but knowing you're a carrier — and taking antibiotics — makes it 20 to 30 times less likely that your baby will contract early-onset disease.

You may wonder why you can't take antibiotics as soon as you receive a positive test, instead of waiting until labour begins. The reason is simple: Taking oral antibiotics in the third trimester isn't effective at preventing the transmission of GBS, because the bacterium can grow back quickly.

How GBS affects labour and baby's first days?: Antibiotics for GBS aren't just for pregnant women with a positive GBS test. If you haven't undergone screening for GBS but fall into a high-risk group, you'll likely receive antibiotics, too. The Centers for

Disease Control and Prevention, the American Academy of Pediatrics, and the American College of Obstetricians and Gynecologists recommend treating women with:

- A positive prenatal GBS culture at 35 to 37 weeks
- A urinary tract infection caused by GBS
- A previous baby with GBS disease
- Fever during labour
- Rupture of membranes 18 hours or more before delivery
- Labour before 37 weeks

If you fall into one of these categories, you'll receive intravenous antibiotics, such as penicillin or ampicillin, when your labour begins. If you're allergic to penicillin and related drugs, you may receive clindamycin or a similar alternative. Doctors generally try to give two doses of antibiotics four hours apart before delivery. If you have a long labour, you may receive additional doses. Medications usually aren't necessary for women who have a Caesarean birth, but it's not necessary to have a Caesarean birth because of GBS.

After delivery, your doctors and nurses will observe your baby to see if he or she needs extra testing or treatment. If there wasn't time to give two doses of antibiotics during labour — and this can happen — there's no need to be concerned. The chance of infection is extremely small, but your doctor may give your baby antibiotics after birth.

Receiving antibiotics for GBS during labour generally means that you'll need to be hooked up to an intravenous (IV) line at some point. Otherwise, being a GBS carrier doesn't change your birth plan. It typically doesn't affect the length of time you and your baby will spend in the hospital. And it doesn't affect your ability to breast-feed safely.

If you had a positive GBS test, you just need to remind the doctor or midwife attending to your delivery when your water breaks or when you arrive at the hospital in labour. Also make sure your labour nurse knows. Don't worry about repeating yourself or appearing overly anxious. Your emphatic reminders will help your doctor or midwife better manage your pregnancy and delivery.

PREGNANCY: SYMPTOMS AND EMOTIONS IN THE THIRD TRIMESTER

The last stage of pregnancy may bring new pregnancy symptoms but relieve earlier ones.

The last few months of pregnancy can be physically and emotionally challenging. Your baby's size and position may make it hard for you to get comfortable. You may be tired of pregnancy and anxious to get it over with. If you've been gearing up for your due date, you may be disappointed to see it come and go uneventfully.

Try to remain positive as you look forward to the end of your pregnancy. Soon you'll hold your baby in your arms! Here's what to expect in the meantime.

Your body: As your baby grows, his or her movements will become more obvious. These exciting sensations are often accompanied by increasing discomfort and other late pregnancy symptoms.

- *Backaches:* As your pregnancy advances, your baby gains weight, while hormones continue to relax the joints between the bones in your pelvic area. These changes can be tough on your back. Hip pain is common, too.

  If you must stand, place one foot on a box or stool. Sit in chairs with good back support. Apply a heating pad or ice pack to the painful area. Ask your partner for a massage. If the back pain doesn't go away or is accompanied by other signs and symptoms, contact your health care provider.

- *Swelling:* Swollen feet and ankles may become an issue at this stage of pregnancy. Your growing uterus puts pressure on the veins that return blood from your feet and legs. Fluid retention and dilated blood vessels may leave your face and eyelids puffy, especially in the morning.

If you have problems with swelling, use cold compresses on the affected areas. Lying down or using a footrest may relieve ankle swelling. It may also help to swim or even stand in a pool.

- *Shortness of breath:* You may get winded easily as your uterus expands beneath your diaphragm, the muscle just below your lungs. This may improve when the baby settles deeper into your pelvis before delivery. In the meantime, practice good posture and sleep on your side. As long as your health care provider says it's OK, aerobic exercise can help relieve this effect of pregnancy, too.

- *Heartburn:* Your growing uterus may push your stomach out of its normal position, which can contribute to heartburn. To keep stomach acid where it belongs, eat small meals and drink plenty of fluids throughout your pregnancy.

- *Spider veins, varicose veins and hemorrhoids:* Increased blood circulation may cause small reddish spots that sprout tiny blood vessels on your face, neck, upper chest or arms — especially if you have fair skin. Varicose veins — blue or reddish lines beneath the surface of the skin — also may appear, particularly in the legs. Hemorrhoids — varicose veins in your rectum — are another possibility.

If you have painful varicose veins, elevate your legs and wear support stockings. To prevent hemorrhoids, include plenty of fiber in your diet and drink lots of fluids.

- *Stretch marks:* You may notice pink, red or purple streaks along your abdomen, breasts, upper arms, buttocks or thighs. Your stretching skin may also be itchy. Moisturisers can help. Although stretch marks can't be prevented, eventually they fade in intensity.

- *Continued breast growth:* By now, you may have an additional 1 to 3 pounds of breast tissue. As delivery approaches, your nipples may start leaking colostrum — the yellowish fluid that will nourish your baby during the first few days of life.

- *Frequent urination:* As your baby moves deeper into your pelvis, you'll feel more pressure on your bladder. You may find yourself urinating more often, even during the night. This extra pressure may also cause you to leak urine — especially when you laugh, cough or sneeze.

Continue to watch for signs of a urinary tract infection, such as urinating even more than usual, burning during urination, fever, abdominal pain or backache. Left untreated, a urinary tract infection may damage your kidneys and trigger preterm labour.

- *Braxton Hicks contractions:* These contractions are warm-ups for the real thing. They're painless and come and go unpredictably. True labour contractions get longer, stronger and closer together. If you're having contractions that concern you, contact your health care provider.

- *Weight gain:* By your due date, you'll probably weigh 25 to 35 pounds more than you did before pregnancy. Your baby accounts for some of the weight gain, but you also need to count the placenta, amniotic fluid, larger breasts and uterus, extra fat stores, and increased blood and fluid volume.

Your emotions: As anticipation grows, fears about childbirth may become more persistent. How much will it hurt? How long will it last? How will I cope?

If you haven't done so already, you may want to take a childbirth class. You'll learn what to expect — and meet other moms-to-be who probably feel the same way you do. Talk with women who've had positive birth experiences, and find out what options you may have for pain relief. Tell yourself that you'll simply do the best you can. There's no right or wrong way to have a baby.

The reality of parenthood may start to sink in as well. You may feel anxious and overwhelmed, especially if this is your first baby. To stay calm, revel in the emotions and sensations of being pregnant.

- Write your thoughts in a journal.
- Listen to soft music.
- Talk to your baby.
- Take photos of your pregnant belly to share with your baby one day.

It also may help to review your decisions about issues such as circumcision and breast-feeding. Knowing how you'll proceed once the baby arrives can give you a greater sense of control.

Appointments with your health care provider: During the third trimester, your health care provider may ask you to come in for more frequent checkups — perhaps every other week beginning at week 32 and every week beginning at week 36.

Like previous visits, your health care provider will check your weight and blood pressure and ask about any signs or symptoms you may be experiencing. You may need screening tests for various conditions, including:

- *Gestational diabetes:* This is a temporary type of diabetes that sometimes develops during pregnancy. Prompt treatment and healthy lifestyle choices can help you manage your blood sugar levels and deliver a healthy baby.

- *Anemia:* Anemia is an abnormally low level of red blood cells or hemoglobin, a protein in red blood cells that contains iron. Severe anemia may slow your baby's growth or trigger preterm labour. To treat anemia, you may need to take iron supplements.

- *Group B strep:* Group B strep is a type of bacteria that may live in your vagina or rectum. It won't make you sick, but it may cause a serious infection for your baby after birth. If you test positive for group B strep, your health care provider may recommend antibiotics while you're in labour.

Your health care provider will also check your baby's size and heart rate. Near the end of your pregnancy, vaginal exams will help your health care provider determine your baby's position inside your uterus. He or she may also check your cervix to see whether it's begun to soften or dilate in preparation for birth.

As your due date approaches, keep asking questions. How can I tell the difference between false labour and the real thing? When do I need to go to the hospital? Could I be too late for an epidural? Remember, there's no silly question. Understanding what's happening can help you have the most positive birth experience.

4

Abnormal Changes in Pregnancy

ECTOPIC PREGNANCY

An ectopic pregnancy is one in which the conceptus (the products of conception—i.e., the placenta, the membranes, and the embryo) implants or attaches itself in a place other than the normal location in the lining of the upper uterine cavity. The site of implantation may be either at an abnormal location within the uterus itself or in an area outside the uterus. Ectopic pregnancies outside the uterine cavity occur about once in every 300 pregnancies. They are one of the major causes of maternal deaths.

Normally an ovum or egg passes from the ovary into the tube, is fertilized in the tube, and moves downward into the uterus. It buries itself in the lining of the upper part of the uterine cavity. It may pass farther down and attach itself to the lining of the mouth of the uterus (the cervix), creating a cervical pregnancy. These are rare and cause severe vaginal bleeding; the conceptus is expelled or discovered within a few months after implantation.

If a conceptus attaches itself to the lower part of the uterine cavity, it is a low implantation. When a low implantation occurs, the placenta grows over the cervical opening, in a formation called a placenta praevia. This causes the woman to bleed, often profusely, through the vagina, because the placenta tears as the cervix begins to open during the latter part of pregnancy.

When the fertilized egg implants in the narrow space or angle of the uterine cavity near the connection of the uterus with the fallopian tube, it is called an angular pregnancy; many angular pregnancies terminate in abortions; others go to term but are complicated because the placenta does not separate properly from the uterine wall after the birth of the baby. An angular pregnancy differs from a cornual pregnancy, which develops in the side of a bilobed or bicornate uterus.

Implantation in the narrow part of the fallopian, or uterine, tube, which lies within the uterine wall, produces what is called an interstitial pregnancy. This occurs in approximately 4 percent of ectopic pregnancies. An interstitial pregnancy gradually stretches the wall of the uterus until—usually between the 8th and 16th week of gestation—the wall ruptures in an explosive manner and there is profuse bleeding into the abdomen.

Most persons associate ectopic pregnancies with tubal pregnancies, because most ectopic pregnancies occur in the uterine tubes.

The tube beyond the uterus has three parts: the isthmus, a narrow section near the uterus; the ampulla, which is wider and more dilatable; and the infundibulum, the flaring, trumpetlike portion of the tube nearest the ovary. A tubal ectopic pregnancy is designated by the area of the tube in which it is implanted. An isthmic pregnancy differs from one in the ampulla or infundibulum because the narrow tube cannot expand. Rupture of the affected tube with profuse intra-abdominal hemorrhage occurs early, usually within eight weeks after conception.

Ampullar pregnancies, which are by far the most common, usually terminate either in a tubal abortion, in which the embryo and the developing afterbirth are expelled through the open end of the tube into the abdomen; by a tubal rupture; or, less commonly, by absorption of the conceptus.

Sometimes the tube ruptures into the tissues attaching it to the wall of the pelvis, producing an intraligamentous pregnancy. Rarely, the embryo is expelled into the abdomen and the afterbirth remains attached to the tube; the embryo lives and grows. Such a condition is referred to as a secondary abdominal pregnancy. Primary abdominal pregnancies, in which the fertilized egg attaches to an abdominal organ, and ovarian pregnancies are rarer still.

It is generally believed, but not proved, that most tubal pregnancies are caused by scars, pockets, kinks, or adhesions in the tubal lining resulting from tubal infections. The infection may have been gonorrhea; it may have occurred after an abortion, after the delivery of a baby, or after a pelvic surgical operation; or it may have been caused by appendicitis. Kinking, scarring, and partial adhesions of the outside of the tube may be the result of inflammation following a pelvic operation or of an abdominal inflammation.

Tubes, defective from birth, may be too small for the passage of the conceptus or may be pocketed or doubled with one tubal half forming a blind pocket. There may be areas in the tubal lining that behave like the lining of the uterus (they show a decidual reaction that is conducive to implantation) so that they offer a favourable spot for the fertilized egg to implant. Pelvic tumours may distort the tube and obstruct it so that the conceptus cannot move downward. Theoretically, endocrine disturbances may delay tubal motility.

Whatever the cause, when a tubal implantation occurs, it may be assumed that either migration of the fertilized egg within the tube was delayed by an extrinsic factor so that the egg grew to the point where it should implant or that the mechanism for implantation within the egg itself was prematurely activated in the tube. One or the other of these causative factors can sometimes be seen when a woman is operated upon for an ectopic pregnancy. In a great number of cases, however, no tube abnormality can be found. There is no satisfactory explanation for most abnormal implantations in the uterus, although defective uterine structure has been noted in some cases.

Primary abdominal and ovarian pregnancies can best be explained by a mechanism in which the fertilized ovum is swept out of the tube by a reverse peristalsis of the tube, but it is quite possible that, in rare instances, the ovum and spermatozoa meet and fertilization and implantation take place within the abdomen.

Ectopic pregnancy is frequently mistaken for other disorders. Typically, but not invariably, the woman who has an ectopic pregnancy in the ampullar part of the tube will have missed one or two menstrual periods. She need not have other symptoms of pregnancy. She has felt enough discomfort in the lower part of her abdomen to lead her to consult a physician. She has had recurrent episodes of rather light, irregular bleeding from the vagina. She has felt weak or faint at times. The signs of pregnancy are not likely to be present, and results of a pregnancy test are more often negative than positive. The physician, on pelvic examination, feels a tender, soft mass in one side of the pelvis. At this stage the differentiation must be made between an ectopic pregnancy and an intrauterine pregnancy with abortion, acute appendicitis, intestinal colic, inflammation of a fallopian tube, and a twisted ovarian tumour. Unless the diagnosis can be made, the patient continues to complain for several more days and then has a sudden severe pain and collapses from brisk bleeding within the abdomen.

Sudden and acute abdominal pain and collapse due to severe hemorrhage are only rarely the first signs that something is amiss. If this does happen, it is usually because implantation has occurred in the isthmic portion of the tube and hemorrhage and tubal rupture occur simultaneously. More frequently, a woman has missed one menstrual period, has a sensation of pelvic pressure, feels that she must urinate, and collapses in the bathroom. She may be unconscious and pulseless from loss of blood when she arrives at the hospital.

Interstitial pregnancies are often mistaken for intrauterine ones, but the patient has pain and may have intermittent vaginal bleeding. After several months she has sudden, severe pain, collapses from a massive intra-abdominal hemorrhage, and may die before surgical help can reach her. Most of the women who die from ectopic pregnancies do so from interstitial ones.

Combined pregnancies, in which there is an ectopic pregnancy and a normal one in the uterus, or a fetus in each tube, have occurred and have compounded the difficulty in making a diagnosis. In a number of instances, the ectopic conceptus has been removed without complications, and the uterine fetus has progressed to term. Not all ectopic pregnancies end with a catastrophic hemorrhage and collapse. In a few instances tubal, abdominal, and broad ligament pregnancies have gone on until a living baby was obtained at the time of operation. In other cases the fetus died and, if very young, was resorbed; in others, when the fetus was larger, death was followed by absorption of the fluid in the sac, and the fetus was gradually converted into a more or less mummified mass. Some ectopic pregnancies of this type have caused no symptoms and have been carried by women for years. Undoubtedly many ectopic pregnancies that are in an early stage when they are expelled emerge through the open end of the uterine tube, are resorbed, and are never recognized.

Once diagnosed, the treatment of ectopic pregnancies outside the uterine cavity is almost always a matter of prompt surgical intervention with proper attention to replacement of blood and fluid.

ABORTION

Abortion is the termination of a pregnancy before the infant can survive outside the uterus. The age at which a fetus is considered viable has not been completely agreed upon. Many obstetricians use either 21 weeks or 400–500 grams (0.9–1.1 pounds) birth weight as the baseline between abortion and premature delivery, because few infants have survived when they weighed less than 500 grams at birth or when the pregnancy was of less than 21 weeks' duration. Generally speaking, the fetus has almost no chance of living if it weighs less than 1,000 grams (2.2 pounds) and if the pregnancy is of less than 24 weeks' duration. In one effort to resolve the matter, the American College of Obstetricians and Gynecologists has defined abortion as the expulsion or extraction of all (complete) or any part (incomplete) of the placenta or membranes, with or without an abortus, before the 20th week (before 134 days) of gestation. Early abortion is an abortion that occurs before the 12th completed week of gestation (84 days); late abortion is an abortion that occurs after the 12th completed week but before the beginning of the 20th week of gestation (85–134 days).

In the past the word abortion usually meant to nonmedical persons the elective interruption of a pregnancy, whereas "miscarriage" indicated a spontaneous expulsion of the uterine contents. The term miscarriage is seldom used medically.

Spontaneous abortion is the expulsion of the products of conception before the 20th week of gestation without deliberate interference. As a general rule, natural causes are responsible for loss of the pregnancy. An induced abortion is the deliberate interruption of a pregnancy by any means before the 20th week of gestation. In medical terminology an abortion may be therapeutic or elective (voluntary). A therapeutic abortion is the interruption of a pregnancy before the 20th week of gestation because it endangers the mother's life or health or because the baby presumably would not be normal. An elective abortion is the interruption of a pregnancy before the 20th week of gestation at the woman's request for reasons other than maternal health or fetal disease. Most abortions in the United States are performed for this reason.

A spontaneous abortion usually passes through several progressive stages. The first stage is a threatened abortion in which a woman, known to be less than 20 weeks pregnant, notices a small amount of bloody discharge from her vagina and, perhaps, a few cramping pains in her uterus. By pelvic examination it is determined that her cervix has not started to open or dilate. Either the symptoms subside or the matter progresses to an inevitable abortion, in which there is increased bleeding, the uterine cramps become more severe, and the cervix, or mouth of the uterus, opens for the expulsion of the uterine contents. An inevitable abortion terminates either as a complete or an incomplete abortion, depending on whether or not all the products of gestation are expelled. The process may start abruptly with pain and profuse bleeding and be over in a few hours, or it may go on for days with only a modest loss of blood. Spontaneous abortions early in pregnancy tend to be complete. When the pregnancy is further advanced, it is more likely to be incomplete. Usually the physician removes the retained tissue in the uterus surgically when there is an incomplete abortion.

If the fetus dies and is retained in the uterus for eight weeks or longer, the condition is referred to as a missed abortion. Women who lose three or more consecutive pregnancies of less than 20 weeks' duration are said to suffer from recurrent abortion. An infected abortion is an abortion associated with infection of the genital organs.

Approximately 15 percent of all clinically evident pregnancies terminate in spontaneous abortion. A much higher rate of early pregnancy loss—more than 40 percent—is believed to occur. Some are lost so early that the woman and her physician are not sure whether she aborted or had a menstrual period that was slightly delayed, particularly heavy, and more painful than usual. The majority occur between the 6th and the 12th week after conception. Modifications in the abortion laws in several countries, including the United States, have greatly increased the number of requested abortions; it is believed that in some areas the number of abortions exceeds that of babies delivered alive.

At least half of all spontaneous first-trimester abortions have been found by karyotyping (examination of chromosome characteristics) to have a chromosomal abnormality. Some of these genetic mistakes are caused by abnormal characteristics carried in the egg or sperm or by the failure of normal rearrangement of the chromosomes to occur after the egg and sperm unite. It has been shown in animals that disturbances in the transportation of the fertilized egg to the uterus may cause premature or delayed implantation of the conceptus; fertilized eggs that are too young or too old tend to abort.

Inadequate secretion of the ovarian hormones estrogen and progesterone, needed for the development of the newly fertilized egg, may cause failure of the lining of the uterus and its secretions to sustain the young embryo. Later, failure of the placenta to take over the hormone-producing function of the ovary may adversely affect the growth of the uterus and its contractility. X rays in large doses, radium, and certain drugs may cause abortion because they damage embryonic tissues. Abnormal development of the mother's uterus may make it impossible for it to retain the pregnancy.

Late abortion is sometimes caused by the weakness of the cervix or by fetal death following knotting of the umbilical cord. Uterine tumours may cause abortion because they increase uterine irritability or create an unfavourable environment for embryonic growth. In most instances in which psychological factors allegedly caused an abortion, examination of the baby and of the afterbirth have shown defects in one or both that had occurred before the mother had suffered her emotional disturbance. Physical injury to the mother is a causative factor in only one in a thousand abortions. Abortions thought to be caused by automobile accidents, falls, kicks, and so forth are often the result of deleterious changes in the fetus and sac that occurred before the injury. Systemic diseases may play a role in causing an abortion. This is particularly true of acute infectious diseases with high fever and bacteria in the bloodstream, or of diseases such as pneumonia, in which there is a marked reduction in the supply of oxygen to the fetus. Heart disease, kidney disease, diabetes, high blood pressure, and other chronic diseases may be associated with premature birth and fetal death after the 21st week but do not ordinarily cause abortions.

Perhaps 3 percent of threatened abortions are prevented by rest and hormonal therapy. Most abortions are inevitable because the fertilized egg is abnormal; these cannot be controlled medically. Many women who suffer from recurrent abortion respond well to treatment; in some of these cases corrective surgery is necessary. An early spontaneous abortion without infection is rarely followed by ill health when the affected person receives proper medical treatment. Infected abortions, many the result of elective interruptions of pregnancy, have caused chronic pelvic distress and, in some cases, sterility.

5

Diet, Exercise and Lifestyle

PREGNANCY AND EXERCISE

Exercise during pregnancy can help you stay in shape and prepare for labour and delivery. But be sure to do it safely.

Pregnancy seems like a perfect time to sit back and relax. You may feel more tired than usual, your back may ache, and your ankles may be swollen. But unless you're experiencing serious complications, sitting around won't help. In fact, pregnancy can be a great time to get active— even if you haven't exercised in a while.

Exercise can help ease or even prevent discomfort, boost your energy level and improve your overall health. Exercise also helps you prepare for labour by increasing your stamina and muscle strength. Being in good shape may even shorten your labour and speed your recovery.

Getting the OK

Before you begin an exercise programme, make sure you have your health care provider's OK. Although exercise during pregnancy is generally good for both mother and baby, you'll need to proceed with caution if you have a history of preterm labour or various medical conditions, including:

- Diabetes
- High blood pressure
- Heart disease

- Placenta previa, a problem with the placenta that can cause excessive bleeding before or during delivery

Pacing it for pregnancy: For most pregnant women, the American College of Obstetricians and Gynecologists recommends at least 30 minutes of moderate exercise on most, if not all, days of the week. But even shorter or less frequent workouts can help you stay in shape and prepare for labour.

Walking is a great exercise for beginners. It provides moderate aerobic conditioning with minimal stress on your joints. Other good choices include swimming and cycling on a stationary bike. Avoid contact sports, scuba diving, exercises that require you to lie flat on your back, and activities that may lead to falls or abdominal injuries.

If you exercised before pregnancy, you can probably continue to work out at the same level while you're pregnant — as long as you're feeling comfortable and your health care provider says it's OK. If you haven't exercised for a while, begin with as little as five minutes of physical activity a day. Build up to 10 minutes, 15 minutes, and so on, until you reach at least 30 minutes a day.

Remember to stretch before and after each workout. Drink plenty of fluids to stay hydrated, and be careful to avoid overheating. No matter how dedicated you are to being in shape, don't exercise to the point of exhaustion.

Staying motivated: You're more likely to stick with an exercise plan if it involves activities you enjoy and fits into your daily schedule. Consider these tips.

- *Start small:* You don't need to join a gym or don expensive workout clothes to get in shape. Just get moving. Try a daily walk through your neighborhood. Vary your route to keep it interesting.

- *Find a partner:* Exercise can be more interesting if you use the time to chat with a friend. Better yet, involve the whole family.

- *Use a headset:* Listen to music or a book on tape, compact disc or MP3 while you exercise. Use lively songs to energise your workout.

- *Try a class:* Many fitness centers and hospitals offer classes designed for pregnant women. Choose one that fits your interests and schedule.
- *Get creative:* Don't limit yourself. Consider hiking, rowing or dancing.
- *Give yourself permission to rest:* Your tolerance for strenuous exercise will decrease as your pregnancy progresses.

Listen to your body: Sometimes the stresses of pregnancy are too much. You may experience various signs or symptoms while you're exercising, including:

- Blurred vision
- Dizziness
- Nausea
- Fatigue
- Shortness of breath
- Headaches
- Chest pain
- Abdominal pain

Don't take any chances. If you experience any of these signs or symptoms, stop what you're doing. If you don't feel better quickly, contact your health care provider.

A healthy choice: Regular exercise can help you cope with the physical changes of pregnancy and build stamina for the challenges ahead. If you haven't been exercising regularly, use pregnancy as your motivation to begin.

PREGNANCY NUTRITION: FOODS TO AVOID

Eating healthy foods is only part of pregnancy nutrition. It's equally important to avoid harmful foods.

You want what's best for your baby. That's why you slice fruit on your fortified breakfast cereal, sneak extra veggies into your favorite recipes and eat yogurt for dessert. But did you know that what you *don't* eat and drink may be just as important as what you do?

Start with the basics. Knowing what to avoid can help you make the healthiest choices for you and your baby.

Seafood: Seafood can be a great source of protein and iron, and the omega-3 fatty acids in many fish can help promote your baby's brain development. However, some fish and shellfish contain potentially dangerous levels of mercury. Too much mercury may damage your baby's developing nervous system. The bigger and older the fish, the more mercury it may contain. Don't eat:

- Swordfish
- Shark
- King mackerel
- Tilefish

So what's safe? Some types of seafood contain little mercury. According to the most recent guidelines from the Food and Drug Administration (FDA), you can safely eat up to 12 ounces a week (two average meals) of:

- Shrimp
- Canned light tuna (Limit albacore tuna and tuna steak to no more than 6 ounces a week.)
- Salmon
- Pollock
- Catfish

In July 2006, a popular consumer magazine raised questions about the safety of any type of canned tuna for pregnant women. The FDA continues to support the safety of up to 12 ounces a week of fish and shellfish that are lower in mercury, including canned light tuna.

To avoid ingesting harmful bacteria or viruses, avoid raw fish and shellfish — especially oysters and clams — and anything caught in polluted water. Refrigerated smoked seafood is also off limits, unless it's an ingredient in a casserole or other cooked dish.

When you cook fish, use the 10-minute rule. Measure the fish at its thickest part and cook for 10 minutes per inch at 450 F. Boil shellfish— such as clams, oysters and shrimp — for four to six minutes.

Meat and poultry: During pregnancy, changes in your metabolism and circulation may increase the risk of bacterial food poisoning. Your reaction may be more severe than if you weren't pregnant. Rarely, your baby may get sick, too.

To prevent food-borne illness, fully cook all meats and poultry before eating. Look for the juices to run clear, but use a meat thermometer to make sure.

Skip medium or rare burgers and sausages. The Escherichia coli (E. coli) bacteria commonly found on the surface of meat may be distributed throughout the whole product during the grinding process. Unless you cook ground meat to an internal temperature of 160 F, you may not raise its internal temperature enough to kill E. coli. Use a meat thermometer to make sure the meat is done.

Be careful with hot dogs and deli meats, too. These are sources of a rare but potentially serious food-borne illness known as listeriosis. Cook hot dogs and heat deli meats until they're steaming hot — or avoid them completely.

Dairy products: Dairy products such as skim milk, mozzarella cheese and cottage cheese can be a healthy part of your diet. But anything containing unpasteurised milk is a no-no. These products may lead to food-borne illness.

Unless these soft cheeses are clearly labeled as being made with pasteurised milk, don't eat:

- Brie
- Feta
- Camembert
- Blue-veined cheeses, such as Roquefort
- Mexican-style cheeses, such as queso blanco, queso fresco, queso de hoja, queso de crema and asadero

Caffeine: During pregnancy, moderate caffeine intake — 200 milligrams or less a day, about the amount in two cups of coffee — seems to have no adverse effects. But that doesn't mean caffeine is free of risks.

Caffeine can cross the placenta and affect your baby's heart rate and breathing. Heavy caffeine intake — 500 milligrams or more a day, about the amount in five cups of coffee — may lower your baby's birth weight and head circumference.

Because of the unknowns, your health care provider may recommend limiting caffeine intake to less than 200 milligrams a day.

Herbal tea: Although herbal tea may be soothing, avoid it unless your health care provider says it's OK. Large amounts of some herbal teas — including peppermint and red raspberry leaf — may cause contractions and increase the risk of miscarriage or preterm labour.

Alcohol: One drink isn't likely to hurt your baby — but no level of alcohol has been proved safe during pregnancy. The safest bet is to avoid alcohol entirely.

Consider the risks. Mothers who drink alcohol have a higher risk of miscarriage and stillbirth. Excessive alcohol consumption may result in fetal alcohol syndrome, which can cause facial deformities, heart problems, low birth weight and mental retardation. Even moderate drinking can impact your baby's brain development.

If you think you might need help to stop drinking alcohol, talk with your health care provider.

PREGNANCY: ESSENTIAL NUTRIENTS

When you're pregnant, eat foods packed with these nutrients.

There's no magical formula for nutrition during pregnancy. Although you'll use an extra 300 calories a day, the basic principles of healthy eating remain the same — plenty of fruits, vegetables and whole grains and leaner sources of protein.

However, a few nutrients do deserve special attention. Here's what tops the list.

Folic acid: This B vitamin helps prevent neural tube defects, serious abnormalities of the brain and spinal cord. Lack of folic acid also increases the risk of preterm delivery, low birth weight and poor fetal growth.

How much you need: 1 milligram (1,000 micrograms) a day before conception and during pregnancy.

Good sources: Fortified cereals are great sources of folic acid. Various fruits and vegetables are other good choices.

Food category	Serving size	Folic acid content
Fortified breakfast cereal	3/4 cup 100 percent fortified ready-to-eat cereal	400 micrograms
Lentils	1/2 cup cooked	180 micrograms
Leafy green vegetables	1/2 cup frozen, cooked or boiled spinach	100 micrograms
Beans and peas	1/2 cup cooked beans	90 to 125 micrograms
Orange juice	3/4 cup	55 micrograms

In addition to healthy food choices, a daily prenatal vitamin — starting at least one month before you get pregnant — is strongly recommended to make sure you're getting enough of this essential nutrient.

Calcium: You and your baby need calcium for strong bones and teeth. Calcium also helps your circulatory, muscular and nervous systems run normally. If there's not enough calcium in your diet, the calcium your baby needs will be taken from your bones.

How much you need: 1,000 milligrams a day.

Good sources: Dairy products are the richest sources of calcium. Many fruit juices and breakfast cereals are fortified with calcium.

Food category	Serving size	Calcium content
Yogurt	1 cup nonfat fruit yogurt	285 to 420 milligrams
Milk	1 cup skim milk	306 milligrams
Salmon	1 3-ounce can pink salmon with bones	181 milligrams
Baked beans	1 cup baked beans	86 to 154 milligrams
Broccoli	1 cup chopped broccoli	41 milligrams

Protein: Protein is crucial for your baby's growth, especially during the second and third trimesters. Protein also repairs your cells as your body changes.

How much you need: At least 60 grams a day.

Good sources: Lean meat, poultry, fish and eggs are great sources of protein. Other options include dried beans and peas, tofu and peanut butter.

Food category	Serving size	Protein content
Fish, poultry, pork or beef	3 ounces (about the size of a deck of cards)	19 to 23 grams
Tofu	1/2 cup firm tofu	20 grams
Peanut butter	2 tablespoons smooth peanut butter	8 grams
Eggs	1 large hard-boiled egg	6 grams

Iron: Your body uses iron to make hemoglobin, a protein in the red blood cells that carries oxygen to your tissues. During pregnancy — when your blood volume expands to accommodate changes in your body and your baby must make his or her entire blood supply — your need for iron nearly doubles.

If you don't get enough iron, you may become fatigued and more susceptible to infections. The risk of preterm delivery and low birth weight is also higher.

How much you need: 27 milligrams of elemental iron a day.

Good sources: Lean red meat, poultry and fish are good sources of iron. Iron-fortified breakfast cereals, nuts and dried fruit are other options.

Food category	Serving size	Iron content
Lean sirloin	3-ounce serving broiled lean sirloin	3 milligrams
Nuts	1/2 cup soy nuts	3.5 milligrams
Tofu	1/2 cup firm tofu	3 milligrams
Spinach	1/2 cup boiled spinach	3 milligrams

Prenatal vitamins typically contain iron. Sometimes, a separate iron supplement is recommended.

The iron from animal products, such as meat, is easiest for the body to absorb. To enhance the absorption of iron from plant sources and supplements, eat the food or take the supplement with a food or beverage high in vitamin C — such as orange juice, tomato juice, cantaloupe, strawberries or tomatoes.

Ask about supplements: Even women who eat healthfully every day may miss out on key nutrients. A daily prenatal vitamin — ideally starting before conception — can help fill any gaps. Your health care provider may recommend special supplements if you follow a strict vegetarian diet or have any chronic health conditions.

Pregnancy: Healthy eating for you and your baby

Pregnant? Healthy eating will keep you feeling good and help your baby thrive.

Eating healthfully during pregnancy is one of the best things you can do for yourself and your baby. After all, the food you eat is your baby's only source of nutrition. Smart choices can help you promote proper growth and development.

Here's help making every bite count.

Grains: Grains provide essential carbohydrates, your body's main source of energy. Many whole grain and enriched products also contain fiber, iron, B vitamins, various minerals and protein. Fortified cereals can help you get enough folic acid.

How much: Choose at least nine servings a day. If that sounds like a lot, relax. It may not be as much as you think.

One serving equals:
- 1 cup cold cereal
- 1/2 cup cooked cereal, pasta or rice
- 1 slice bread
- 1/2 English muffin
- 1/2 small bagel
- 6 crackers

Trade sugary cereal and white bread for whole-grain cereals, brown rice, whole-wheat pasta and whole-grain bread. Feature wild rice or barley in soups, stews, casseroles and salads. Look for products that list whole grains first in the ingredients list (such as whole-wheat flour, not simply wheat flour). Some packages also feature the "Whole Grain" stamp from the Whole Grains Council.

Fruits and vegetables: Fruits and vegetables provide various vitamins and minerals, as well as fiber to aid digestion. Vitamin C, found in many fruits and vegetables, helps you absorb iron. It also promotes healthy gums and other tissues for both you and your baby. Dark green vegetables have vitamin A, iron and folic acid — other important nutrients during pregnancy.

How much: Choose three or more servings of fruit and four or more servings of veggies a day. It's easy! Top your cereal with slices of fresh fruit. Make a veggie pizza. Sneak extra vegetables into your casserole.

One serving equals:
- 1 medium-sized piece of fruit
- 1/2 cup fresh, frozen or canned fruit
- 1/4 cup dried fruit
- 1 cup raw, leafy vegetables
- 1/2 cup cooked or other raw vegetables
- 3/4 cup fruit or vegetable juice
- 1 small baked potato

If you're tired of the standard apples, oranges, green beans and corn, branch out. Try apricots, mango, pineapple, sweet potatoes, winter squash or asparagus.

Meat, eggs and beans: Foods in this group have plenty of protein, as well as B vitamins and iron.

How much: Choose at least three servings of protein-rich foods a day. Lean meat is a great choice. Eat peanut butter toast for breakfast. Make scrambled eggs or an omelet for dinner. Add chickpeas or black beans to your salad. Snack on a handful of soy nuts.

One serving equals:
- 3 ounces of cooked lean meat, poultry or fish (about the size of a deck of cards)
- 1/2 cup cooked dried beans

- 1 egg
- 1/2 cup tofu
- 1/3 cup nuts
- 2 tablespoons peanut butter

Sex during pregnancy: An unnecessary taboo?

Is it OK to have sex during pregnancy? Will it hurt the baby? Learn what's OK — and what's not OK — when you're pregnant.

If you want to get pregnant, you have sex. No surprises there. But what about sex while you're pregnant? The answers aren't always as clear. Here's what you need to know about sex during pregnancy.

Is it OK to have sex during pregnancy?: As long as your pregnancy is proceeding normally, you can have sex as often as you like. But you may not always want to. At first, hormonal fluctuations, fatigue and nausea may sap your sexual desire. During the second trimester, increased blood flow to your sexual organs and breasts may rekindle your desire for sex. But by the third trimester, weight gain, back pain and other symptoms may once again dampen your enthusiasm for sex.

Can sex cause a miscarriage?: Many couples worry that sex during pregnancy will cause a miscarriage, especially in the first trimester. But sex isn't a concern. Early miscarriages are usually related to chromosomal abnormalities or other problems in the developing baby — not to anything you do or don't do.

Does sex harm the baby?: The baby is protected by the amniotic fluid in your uterus, as well as the mucous plug that blocks the cervix throughout most of your pregnancy. Your partner's penis won't touch the baby.

Are any sexual positions off-limits during pregnancy?: As your pregnancy progresses, experiment to find the most comfortable positions. There's just one caveat. Avoid lying flat on your back during sex. If your uterus compresses the veins in the back of your abdomen, you may feel lightheaded or nauseous.

What about oral sex?: If you have oral sex, make sure your partner does not blow air into your vagina. Rarely, a burst of air may block a blood vessel (air embolism) — which could be a life-threatening condition for you and the baby.

Can orgasms trigger premature labour?: Orgasms can cause uterine contractions. But these contractions are different from the contractions you'll feel during labour. Research indicates that if you have a normal pregnancy, orgasms — with or without intercourse — don't lead to premature labour or premature birth.

Are there times when sex should be avoided?: Although most women can safely have sex throughout pregnancy, sometimes it's best to be cautious.

- *Preterm labour:* Exposure to the prostaglandins in semen may cause contractions — which could be worrisome if you're at risk of preterm labour.
- *Vaginal bleeding:* Sex is not recommended if you have unexplained vaginal bleeding.
- *Problems with the cervix:* If your cervix begins to open prematurely (cervical incompetence), sex may pose a risk of infection.
- *Problems with the placenta:* If your placenta partly or completely covers your cervical opening (placenta previa), sex could lead to bleeding and preterm labour.
- *Multiple babies:* If you're carrying two or more babies, your doctor may advise you not to have sex late in pregnancy — although researchers have not identified any relationship between sex and preterm labour in twins.

Should my partner use a condom?: Exposure to sexually transmitted diseases during pregnancy increases the risk of infections that can affect your pregnancy and your baby's health. If you have a new sexual partner during pregnancy, use a condom when you have sex.

What if I don't want to have sex?: That's OK. There's more to a sexual relationship than intercourse. Share your needs and concerns with your partner in an open and loving way. If sex is difficult, unappealing or off-limits, try cuddling, kissing or massage.

After the baby is born, how soon can I have sex?: Whether you give birth vaginally or by C-section, your body will need time to heal. Many doctors recommend waiting six weeks before resuming intercourse. This allows time for your cervix to close and any tears or a repaired episiotomy to heal.

If you're too sore or exhausted to even think about sex, maintain intimacy in other ways. Share short phone calls throughout the day or occasional soaks in the tub. When you're ready to have sex, take it slow— and use a reliable method of contraception.

WORKING DURING PREGNANCY

Working during your pregnancy isn't easy. Consider these tips on how to battle morning sickness, fatigue and other physical discomforts at the workplace.

If you're like most pregnant women, it's perfectly safe for you to continue working during your pregnancy. However, just being pregnant can present challenges. After all, your body works nonstop for nine months to create and nurture a baby. Factor in the demands of your job with all the related effects of pregnancy — from nausea and fatigue to back pain and swollen feet — and you can easily feel worn out.

Stay healthy and productive on the job by learning how to alleviate some common discomforts of pregnancy and understanding when occupational duties might jeopardise your pregnancy.

Easing nausea and vomiting: It may be called "morning" sickness, but the queasiness you feel during pregnancy — especially during the first trimester — can hit at just about any time of the day or night.

To help ease nausea when you're on the job:

- *Avoid nausea triggers:* Certain foods and odors can aggravate nausea during pregnancy. That double latte you craved every morning before pregnancy or the smell of foods reheated in the break room microwave may now make your stomach flip-flop. Once you identify things that trigger your nausea, do your best to steer clear of these odors.

- *Eat snacks and light meals:* Crackers and other bland food can be lifesavers when you start to feel nauseated. Keep a stash in your desk drawer at work. Snacking can keep your stomach from becoming completely empty or too full — two conditions that can make nausea worse.
- *Drink plenty of fluids:* Your body needs more water in early pregnancy. If you don't drink enough fluid, nausea can become worse. A good goal is six to eight 8-ounce glasses throughout the day.
- *Get enough sleep:* The more tired you are, the more nauseated you can become. Allow yourself extra time in the morning to get ready for work to avoid rushing around — something else that can trigger nausea.

If you experience severe, prolonged bouts of morning sickness, and simple measures such as these don't help, tell your doctor.

Handling fatigue: Being pregnant, you might feel tired much of the time, especially during the first and third trimesters and even more so after a long day at work.

Fatigue is your body's way of telling you to slow down, but this can be tough during the workday. To make it through the day, try the following:

- *Take short, frequent breaks:* Regular rest periods can improve your productivity, especially if fatigue interferes with your ability to concentrate or make decisions. Getting up and moving around for a few minutes can reinvigorate you. Spending a few minutes during your lunch hour or break time with the lights off, your eyes closed and your feet up also can help you recharge.
- *Rethink your schedule:* Recognise that your energy level fluctuates throughout the workday. If you're exhausted by the afternoon, get your toughest or high-concentration tasks done earlier in the day. If it takes you longer to get charged up in the morning, put off energy-draining chores until the afternoon. If it's an option in your workplace, explore the possibility of flexible work hours to take advantage of the times during the day when your energy level is high.

- *Cut back on commitments and activities outside of work:* This can allow you to get more rest when your workday is over. If you have a physically demanding job, it's even more important to take it easy when you're not working.
- *Be active when you can:* Although the last thing you may feel like doing at the end of a long day is exercising, it may help boost your energy level. Take a walk in the evenings after you get home from work or look into a prenatal fitness class — provided you have the OK from your doctor to do so.
- *Accept help from others:* During work hours, don't be too proud to accept help and support from your co-workers. After work, you may be used to cleaning your house, mowing the lawn and running errands. But to get in extra rest time, consider hiring services to do cleaning or yardwork. Also look into online shopping and home deliveries to gain extra time.
- *Go to bed at a reasonable hour:* If you're tired by 7 p.m., then turn in for the night.

Staying comfortable: Carrying around a growing baby can make everyday activities like sitting, standing, bending and lifting uncomfortable on the job.

Moving around every few hours can ease muscle tension and help prevent fluid buildup in your legs and feet. Empty your bladder frequently to help relieve pressure. And try these other strategies to make yourself comfortable throughout your workday.

Sitting: If you have an office job, the chair you sit in is important. While the weight in your body is increasing and shifting your posture, it helps to have a seat you can adjust for height and tilt. Adjustable armrests, a firm seat and back cushions, and good lower back support can make long hours of sitting much easier.

If your office chair doesn't have these adjustment options, you can improvise. Use a small pillow or a specially designed cushion to provide extra support for your back. Put your feet up on a footrest — or your wastebasket or a box — to take pressure off your lower back and help reduce swelling in your feet.

Standing: During pregnancy, increased dilation of your blood vessels can cause blood to pool in your legs with prolonged periods of standing. This can lead to pain, dizziness or even fainting.

Standing also puts pressure on your back. If standing is part of your job, put one of your feet up on a box or a low stool to take pressure off your back and decrease blood pooling. Switch feet every so often. You also might find it helps to wear support hose, which can improve the circulation in your legs. Wear comfortable shoes and take frequent breaks to rest your legs. If your job requires that you stand four or more hours each day, tell your doctor. If he or she has concerns, you might need to modify your job duties or stop working earlier in your pregnancy.

Bending and lifting: To prevent or ease back pain, follow proper form when bending and lifting. Check with your doctor about recommendations for lifting — in some circumstances, you might be advised to avoid heavy lifting during your pregnancy. Even if you're lifting something that's not too heavy, keep in mind that there's a right way and a wrong way to lift.

Keeping stress under control: Stress on the job can inspire you to push hard and achieve many goals. But it can also exhaust you and take away the time and energy you need to care for yourself and your unborn baby.

It may be impossible to eliminate work-related stress, but you can do your best to minimise it. Talk out problems with a supportive co-worker, friend or spouse. Or your doctor might be able to refer you to a support group that can help you deal with stress before it affects your well-being.

Maintaining a good sense of humor and a positive outlook also can help. Surround yourself with positive, not negative people. Focus on the big picture. When you feel yourself getting angry or upset as a result of stress, stop and ask yourself if you can do anything to change the situation. If not, you may just need to let it go.

Learning and practicing some relaxation exercises also can help you release pressure that may build up during the course of a day. Yoga classes designed for pregnant women offer a unique chance to practice relaxation along with strengthening exercises.

Taking proper job precautions: Certain working conditions may increase your risk of complications during pregnancy, especially if you're at risk of complications for other reasons. These activities and conditions include:

- Heavy, repetitive lifting
- Prolonged standing
- Heavy vibrations, such as from large machines
- Long, stressful commutes to and from work
- Exposure to harmful substances

Other job conditions also may be cause for concern. Frequent shift changes, for instance, may make it hard for you to get the proper rest. A hot work environment may decrease your stamina and ability to perform strenuous physical tasks. Activities that require agility and good balance may become more difficult later in pregnancy.

If any of these issues apply to you, mention them to your doctor. He or she will be able to tell you if you need to take any special precautions or modify your work duties. Your doctor can also make specific recommendations throughout the various stages of your pregnancy and, if needed, provide documents for your employer explaining any work restrictions you might need.

6

Prenatal Care and Testing

An adequate maternal diet is necessary to ensure proper fetal development as well as to maintain the health of the mother. As discussed above, the physiological adjustments of a pregnant woman's body are significant, and nutritional requirements increase as a result. Many physicians recommend that pregnant women also take a prenatal vitamin to ensure adequate vitamin intake. Prenatal vitamins contain a variety of vitamins and minerals, including calcium, folic acid, and iron.

In addition to an awareness of the substances that are of benefit during pregnancy, a knowledge of which substances are harmful and should be avoided is equally important. Alcohol has been found to be teratogenic (causing developmental malformations in the fetus). Intake of large to moderate quantities of alcohol during pregnancy is responsible for fetal alcohol syndrome, which is characterized by impaired growth and development, facial abnormalities, cardiac defects, and skeletal and joint malformations. The effects of limited intake of alcohol are not as well known, but avoidance of any amount of alcohol throughout pregnancy is recommended. Smoking of tobacco during pregnancy is believed to lower the birth weight of the fetus and is also associated with placenta praevia, abruptio placentae, and elevated maternal blood pressure. Sudden infant death syndrome, delayed mental development in childhood, and spontaneous abortion also have been linked to smoking. Limiting the use of caffeine also is encouraged. While not believed to have teratogenic effects, excessive caffeine intake may account for low birth weight in infants. Maternal exposure to high levels of air pollution has also been linked to low infant birth weight. Over-the-counter medications as well as prescription drugs can adversely affect fetal development and should not be taken unless a health-care provider is consulted.

ULTRASOUND

The use of high-frequency sound waves to produce a graphic image of the growing fetus—ultrasonography—is becoming a ubiquitous tool in prenatal medicine, furnishing information on the morphological and functional status of the fetus. It is commonly used to estimate the gestational age of the fetus, identify fetal number, assess growth, determine fetal heart activity, and provide a general survey of fetal anatomy. The presentation of the fetus and placenta and the volume of amniotic fluid also can be determined using ultrasound. In most European countries an ultrasound scan is routinely included in obstetric examinations, but, although it is widely used in the United States and Canada, its inclusion in standard prenatal evaluations has not been recommended. This reluctance is based on the lack of clear evidence that this procedure has no negative effects. Theoretical risks are involved because of the invasive nature of this technique (i.e., sound waves are reflected off tissues). Studies to date, however, have revealed no evidence of tissue damage when diagnostic ultrasound is used, and the benefits of this procedure seem to outweigh the risks.

Amniocentesis

In the procedure of amniocentesis, amniotic fluid is aspirated (withdrawn) from the uterus by a needle inserted through a woman's abdomen, using ultrasound to circumnavigate the fetus and placenta. Spinal cord defects and a host of genetic abnormalities such as Down syndrome and autosomal recessive diseases such as Tay-Sachs disease and cystic fibrosis can be screened for by amniocentesis. It can also be used to determine the sex of the fetus and identify sex-linked diseases. Not all birth defects, however, can be detected by this procedure. This test is generally performed about the 16th week of pregnancy, and results take several weeks to obtain. Of the potential risks associated with this procedure, the most significant one is that of fetal loss, which may result from disruption of the placenta.

Chorionic villi sampling

The technique of retrieving a sample of villi from the chorion (outer embryonic membrane) within the uterus is similar to amniocentesis but can be carried out much earlier in pregnancy, between the 8th and 12th week of gestation. The test can be performed through either the abdomen or the vagina and cervix. The latter technique is carried out using ultrasonic visualization, and a thin catheter is inserted through the vagina into the uterus; a sample of villi from the chorion is then extracted and examined. If unfavourable results are received, termination of the pregnancy can be accomplished at an earlier stage than would be possible with amniocentesis. This procedure does carry a slightly higher risk of fetal loss than does amniocentesis, possibly because it is carried out at an earlier stage in fetal development. With this technique there is also concern that fetal limb reduction or malformation may result, but reports are inconclusive.

Alpha-fetoprotein screening

Shed by the yolk sac and fetal liver, alpha-fetoprotein can be used to screen for neural tube defects such as anencephaly and spina bifida (developmental abnormality in which spinal cord is not fully enclosed). The measurement of elevated levels of alpha-fetoprotein in a woman's blood between the 16th and 18th weeks of pregnancy are associated with this abnormality. Because other circumstances such as multiple pregnancies, underestimation of gestational age, and fetal death are associated with high levels of alpha-fetoprotein, ultrasound should be used to help rule out these different causes. Abnormally low levels of alpha-fetoprotein have been linked to a significant incidence of Down syndrome. A high rate of false-positive results is associated with this test, and so it is not recommended routinely. This procedure has been reserved primarily for those women with a family history of neural tube defects.

PREGNANCY TESTS

Home pregnancy tests are very accurate after the first day of your missed period. If you get a positive result on a home pregnancy test, you should schedule an appointment with your doctor right away. An ultrasound will be used to confirm and date your pregnancy.

Pregnancy is diagnosed by measuring the body's levels of human chorionic gonadotropin (hCG). Also referred to as the pregnancy hormone, hCG is produced upon implantation. However, it may not be detected until after you miss a period.

After you miss a period, hCG levels increase rapidly. hCG is detected through either a urine or a blood test.

Urine tests may be provided at a doctor's office, and they're the same as the tests you can take at home.

Blood tests can be performed in a laboratory. hCG blood tests are about as accurate as home pregnancy tests. The difference is that blood tests may be ordered as soon as six days after ovulation.

The sooner you can confirm you're pregnant, the better. An early diagnosis will allow you to take better care of your baby's health. Get more information on pregnancy tests, such as tips for avoiding a "false negative" result.

PREGNANCY AND VAGINAL DISCHARGE

An increase in vaginal discharge is one of the earliest signs of pregnancy. Your production of discharge may increase as early as one to two weeks after conception, before you've even missed a period.

As your pregnancy progresses, you'll continue to produce increasing amounts of discharge. The discharge will also tend to become thicker and occur more frequently. It's usually heaviest at the end of your pregnancy.

During the final weeks of your pregnancy, your discharge may contain streaks of thick mucus and blood. This is called "the bloody show." It can be an early sign of labor. You should let your doctor know if you have any bleeding.

Normal vaginal discharge, or leukorrhea, is thin and either clear or milky white. It's also mild-smelling.

If your discharge is yellow, green, or gray with a strong, unpleasant odor, it's considered abnormal. Abnormal discharge can be a sign of an infection or a problem with your pregnancy, especially if there's redness, itching, or vulvar swelling.

If you think you have abnormal vaginal discharge, let your healthcare provider know immediately. Learn more about vaginal discharge during pregnancy.

PREGNANCY AND URINARY TRACT INFECTIONS (UTIS)

Urinary tract infections (UTIs) are one of the most common complications women experience during pregnancy. Bacteria can get inside a woman's urethra, or urinary tract, and can move up into the bladder. The fetus puts added pressure on the bladder, which can cause the bacteria to be trapped, causing an infection.

Symptoms of a UTI usually include pain and burning or frequent urination. You may also experience:

- cloudy or blood-tinged urine
- pelvic pain
- lower back pain
- fever
- nausea and vomiting

Nearly 18 percent of pregnant women develop a UTI. You can help prevent these infections by emptying your bladder frequently, especially before and after sex. Drink plenty of water to stay hydrated. Avoid using douches and harsh soaps in the genital area. Contact your healthcare provider if you have symptoms of a UTI. Infections during pregnancy can be dangerous because they increase the risk of premature labor.

When caught early, most UTIs can be treated with antibiotics that are effective against bacteria but still safe for use during pregnancy. Follow the advice here to prevent UTIs before they even start.

CHOOSING YOUR HEALTH CARE PROVIDER FOR PREGNANCY

Whether this is your first pregnancy or your fifth pregnancy, finding the right health care provider can make a big difference in your experience. The person you choose for your health care during pregnancy can make a big difference in the type of childbirth you have. The nature of your pregnancy — determined by your age, the outcomes of your past pregnancies, and health conditions that make pregnancy and childbirth particularly risky for you — may dictate which type of health care provider is best for you. But your personal preferences matter, too. In the United States, doctors deliver about 90 percent of babies, while midwives deliver about 8 percent. In Europe, by contrast, midwives assist at more than 70 percent of normal vaginal births. Before picking your pregnancy care provider, consider all of your options — family physicians, obstetricians, maternal-fetal medicine specialists and midwives.

Where to start

Finding the right health care provider for your pregnancy and childbirth can be a daunting process. To identify potential providers:

- Ask family and friends for recommendations.
- Consult with your regular doctor and other medical professionals.
- Contact your county medical society for a list of the providers in your area.
- Contact the hospital you prefer and find out who its maternity care providers are.

As you study your options, consider these questions:

- Is the health care provider's office a convenient distance from your home or work?
- Can the health care provider deliver your baby in the place you want to give birth — at a particular hospital or birthing center?

- Does the health care provider work in a solo or group practice? If it's a group practice, can you usually see your chosen health care provider or will you see all members of the group?
- Who will replace your health care provider if he or she isn't available in an emergency or when your labour begins?
- How much do the health care provider's services cost? Is the cost covered by your insurance company?
- What level of expertise does your pregnancy require? Will your health care provider meet that need?
- How much do you value the opportunity for your health care provider to serve the entire family?

Family physicians: Primary care for all ages

Family physicians provide care for the whole family through all stages of life, including pregnancy and birth. They have training in various fields of medicine, including obstetrics, pediatrics, internal medicine, gynecology and surgery. Training and experience qualify them to manage most pregnancies, including minor surgical procedures for vaginal delivery. Some perform Caesarean births, but most do not.

Family physicians may work solo, or they may be part of a larger group practice that includes nurses and other medical professionals. They're usually associated with a hospital where they can perform deliveries.

Advantages	Issues to consider
May already know you — and your family and medical history	May refer you to a specialist in obstetrics if you've had problems with a previous pregnancy
May treat your pregnancy as part of the larger picture of your general health and well-being	May refer you to a specialist if you have diabetes, high blood pressure, heart disease or another medical problem that may complicate your pregnancy
Can continue to treat you and your baby after birth	May not be available at the time of your delivery

You might choose a family physician if:

- You and your doctor don't foresee any problems with your pregnancy
- You want your doctor to be involved with all members of your family
- You want continuity in care from prenatal appointments throughout childhood and beyond

Obstetrician-gynecologists: Traditional caregivers for pregnancy and birth

Doctors who specialise in obstetrics and gynecology are commonly referred to as ob-gyns. Besides providing prenatal care and delivering babies, they specialise in the care of women in general, overseeing prevention and treatment of conditions affecting a woman's reproductive organs, breasts and sexual function.

Because of their emphasis on women's health, ob-gyns serve as the main health care provider for many women. They're trained to handle all phases of pregnancy, from preconception planning to postpartum recovery.

Ob-gyns often work in a group practice that may include recent graduates from medical school (residents), nurses, certified nurse-midwives, physician assistants, dietitians and social workers. They may be based in a hospital or clinic.

Advantages	Issues to consider
May already know you — and your gynecologic history	May refer you to a maternal-fetal specialist if you have an extremely high-risk pregnancy
Will be able to continue treating you if problems or complications arise during pregnancy	May not be available at the time of your delivery
Can perform episiotomy, forceps delivery or Caesarean birth	

You might choose an ob-gyn if:

- You have a high-risk pregnancy. You may be high risk if you're over age 35 or you develop diabetes (gestational diabetes) or high blood pressure (preeclampsia) during pregnancy.

- You're carrying twins, triplets or more.
- You have a pre-existing medical condition, such as diabetes, high blood pressure or an autoimmune disorder.
- You want the reassurance that if a problem does arise — such as the need for medical interventions or a Caesarean birth — you won't need to be transferred to a different care provider.

Maternal-fetal medicine specialists: Advanced care for high-risk pregnancies

These doctors, also called perinatologists or high-risk obstetricians, are trained in the care of very high-risk pregnancies. They concentrate exclusively on pregnancy and the unborn child, dealing with the most severe complications that arise. When women with major medical problems become pregnant, their physicians often consult with maternal-fetal medicine specialists in order to optimise care for both the mother and her fetus. Most women don't need the services of a maternal-fetal medicine specialist because most pregnancies are fairly routine.

Maternal-fetal medicine specialists often work as part of a group practice, functioning mainly as consultants rather than primary obstetric care providers. They're often associated with a hospital, university or clinic.

Advantages	Issues to consider
Will be familiar with the complications of pregnancy and adept at recognizing abnormalities	Tend to be less directly involved with their patients than are family physicians, ob-gyns and midwives, although this isn't always true
Will be familiar with the newest approaches to diagnosing and treating obstetric problems	Rarely serve as the primary health care provider for a pregnant woman

You might choose a maternal-fetal medicine specialist if:

- You have a severe medical condition complicating your

pregnancy, such as an infectious disease, heart disease, kidney disease or cancer

- You've previously had severe pregnancy complications or recurrent pregnancy losses
- You have a complicated family medical history, which may require your baby to undergo sophisticated prenatal diagnostic techniques or interventions, such as chorionic villus sampling or fetal surgery
- You're a known carrier of a severe genetic condition that may be passed on to your baby
- Your baby has been diagnosed before birth with a medical condition, such as spina bifida

Midwives: Attentive caregivers in low-risk pregnancies

Midwives provide preconception, maternity and postpartum care for women at low risk of complications during pregnancy. Throughout much of the world, midwives are the traditional care providers for women during pregnancy. In the United States, the use of midwives is steadily increasing. In general, midwives follow the principle that pregnancy and birth are normal, healthy, personal events until proven otherwise. As a result, midwives generally take a lower-tech approach than obstetricians and other doctors typically do.

Midwives vary in the amount of formal training they've received and the services they offer. Midwives are often classified according to their training:

- *Certified nurse-midwives:* These are registered nurses who have completed advanced training in obstetrics and gynecology and have graduated from an accredited nurse-midwifery programme. They are certified by the American College of Nurse-Midwives (ACNM), for which they must pass several exams. Certified nurse-midwives are licensed in all 50 states and the District of Columbia. Some can prescribe medications. Most can recommend diet, exercise and lifestyle changes.
- *Direct-entry midwives:* These midwives don't have a nursing degree but may be trained in other areas of health

care. They may have training through self-study, apprenticeship, a midwifery school or a college- or university-based programme separate from nursing. They may be licensed, certified or neither. Different states have different licensing requirements. Some states have very strict standards. Others don't regulate midwives at all.

- *Certified midwives:* These direct-entry midwives are certified by the ACNM, for which they must pass the same exams required of certified nurse-midwives. This is a fairly new certification and is currently licensed only in the state of New York. However, other states and midwifery organizations may use the same designation for individuals whom they have licensed. Although this may sound confusing, most certified midwives are happy to explain their certification.

- *Certified professional midwives:* These direct-entry midwives have been certified by the North American Registry of Midwives, an international certification agency created by the Midwives Alliance of North America.

- *Lay midwives:* These caregivers are uncertified or unlicensed midwives who generally have had only informal training.

Most midwives in the United States today are certified nurse-midwives or certified midwives.

Midwives may practice solo but often are part of a group practice, such as a team of obstetric care providers. Most midwives are associated with an ob-gyn in case problems occur. The majority of certified nurse-midwives attend births in a hospital or birthing center. Direct-entry midwives are more likely to deliver at home.

If you're considering a midwife, check to see that he or she has a backup arrangement with a hospital so that you'll have access to obstetric skills and equipment in case of pregnancy or birthing problems. If you're not giving birth in a hospital, create an emergency plan that includes such details as the name and number of your midwife's backup doctor, the hospital you'll be taken to, and how you'll get there.

Advantages	Issues to consider
May offer a more natural, less regimented approach to pregnancy and childbirth	May refer you to a specialist in obstetrics if complications develop during your pregnancy
May be able to provide greater individual attention during pregnancy	Can't perform Caesarean births and may not be licensed to administer drugs or anesthesia, if the need arises
Is more likely to be present during labour and delivery than is a doctor.	

You might choose a midwife if:

- You're free of health problems and you expect to have a low-risk pregnancy
- You want someone who can spend a significant amount of time discussing your pregnancy with you
- You prefer a more personalised approach to the birthing process
- You desire a less regimented birthing process
- You desire fewer interventions

Who is right for you?

In the end, it's most important to find someone you can rely on and confide in over the next nine months.

As you meet a potential health care provider, think about these issues:

- Does he or she listen to your concerns and provide helpful answers to your questions?
- Does he or she seem open to and comfortable with your philosophy regarding pregnancy and childbirth?
- Will he or she keep you informed and allow you to participate as you wish in medical decisions affecting you and your baby?

Choose someone you trust to safely guide you and your baby through the birthing process. Then, remember that you chose your health care provider for a reason, and allow him or her to give you the best possible care.

PRENATAL TESTING: COMMON SCREENING AND DIAGNOSTIC TESTS

Along with feelings of excitement and joy, pregnancy often brings moments of doubt and anxiety. It's natural to be concerned about your baby's health or what the future holds. If you're interested in prenatal testing, ask your health care provider which tests might be appropriate for you. Here are the basics on the most common prenatal screening tests.

First trimester screen

What it is? : A two-step screening. First, a maternal blood test for two normal first-trimester proteins. Second, nucal translucency ultrasound to measure a region under the skin behind the baby's neck.

When it's done? Between the 11th and 14th weeks of pregnancy.

How it's done? A blood sample is taken from the mother's arm. Ultrasound takes fetal measurements.

What the results may tell you? Whether the baby has an increased risk of Down syndrome. May help detect certain heart defects or skeletal problems.

Follow-up: Because false positive results are possible, other tests — such as amniocentesis or chorionic villus sampling — may be needed to confirm or rule out a diagnosis.

Quad marker screen

What it is? Maternal blood test for four substances that normally come from a baby's blood, brain, spinal fluid and amniotic fluid.

When it's done? Between the 15th and 20th weeks of pregnancy. Offered to women who did not complete first-trimester screening.

How it's done? A blood sample is taken from the mother's arm.

What the results may tell you? Whether the baby has an increased risk of certain developmental or chromosomal disorders, such as spina bifida or Down syndrome.

Follow-up: One in 20 women have false positive results, so a repeat quad marker screen, an ultrasound or other diagnostic tests may be needed.

Ultrasound

What it is? Sound waves are used to create an image of the baby and the surrounding structures.

When it's done? Between the 18th and 20th weeks of pregnancy.

How it's done? Sound waves from a transducer moved over the mother's abdomen are converted into images on a monitor.

What the results may tell you? Whether the baby's growth and development are on target. Can identify various congenital abnormalities.

Follow-up: Advanced ultrasound and other tests may be needed. Some abnormalities can be treated prenatally.

If the results of a screening test are positive or worrisome, your health care provider may recommend a more invasive diagnostic test. Here are the basics on the most common prenatal diagnostic tests.

Amniocentesis

What it is? A sample of the amniotic fluid is checked for specific genetic problems.

When it's done? After the 15th week of pregnancy.

How it's done? A sample of amniotic fluid is withdrawn from the mother's abdomen with an ultrasound-guided needle.

What the results may tell yo? Can identify chromosomal abnormalities and certain genetic problems, such as Down syndrome and spina bifida.

Possible safety concerns: One in 200 risk of miscarriage when done before the 24th week of pregnancy.

Chorionic villus sampling (CVS)

What it is? A sample of the placenta is tested for genetic abnormalities.

When it's done? Between the 9th and 14th weeks of pregnancy.

How it's done? Guided by ultrasound, a needle is inserted in the uterus or a thin tube is threaded through the cervix and a sample of placental tissue is removed.

What the results may tell yo? Can identify chromosomal abnormalities and some specific genetic problems earlier than amniocentesis.

Possible safety concerns: One in 100 risk of miscarriage.

Percutaneous umbilical blood sampling (PUBS)

What it is? A sample of the baby's blood is tested for genetic problems or infections.

When it's done? After the 18th week of pregnancy.

How it's done? A blood sample is taken from the vein in the umbilical cord through a needle inserted in the mother's abdomen. Ultrasound helps locate the vein.

What the results may tell yo? Can identify sickle cell anemia, hemophilia, anemia, Rh disease and various other conditions.

Possible safety concerns: Two in 100 risk of miscarriage.

Third trimester prenatal care

At the end of your pregnancy, you'll see your health care provider more often. Here's the lowdown on your final prenatal visits. Prenatal care continues until delivery. Your health care provider will continue to monitor your blood pressure and weight, as well as your baby's heartbeat and movements. During the last month of pregnancy, expect weekly checkups.

Testing for group B strep

Most pregnant women are screened for group B streptococcus (GBS) during the third trimester. GBS is a common bacterium that's usually harmless in adults — but babies who become infected with GBS can become critically ill. If a swab from your vagina and rectal area tests positive for GBS, you'll probably be given intravenous antibiotics during labour to protect your baby from the bacterium.

Resuming vaginal exams

As your due date approaches, your checkups may include vaginal exams. Your health care provider may:

- *Check the baby's position:* During a vaginal exam, your health care provider can feel your baby's head in your lower abdomen or at the top of the birth canal. If your baby is positioned headfirst, you're good to go. If your baby is positioned rump-first or feet-first (breech), your health care provider may recommend trying to turn the baby by applying pressure to your abdomen. This procedure is called an external version. If your baby remains in a breech position, you may need a Caesarean delivery.

- *Detect cervical changes:* As your body prepares for birth, your cervix will begin to soften, open (dilate) and thin (efface). Progress is expressed in centimeters (cm) and percentages. For example, your cervix may be 3 cm dilated and 30 percent effaced. When you're ready to push your baby out, your cervix will be 10 cm dilated and 100 percent effaced.

Resist the temptation to put much stock in these numbers. Cervical changes can help your health care provider determine how difficult it would be to induce your labour, but these numbers can't predict spontaneous labour. You may be dilated to 3 cm for weeks — or you may go into labour without any dilation or effacement at all.

Keep asking questions

You may have plenty of questions as your due date approaches. Is it OK to have sex? How will I know when I'm in labour? What's the best way to manage the pain? Ask away! Also discuss a birthing plan with your health care provider. Feeling prepared can help calm your nerves before delivery.

How to get pregnant

Some couples seem to get pregnant simply by talking about it. For others, it takes more effort. Here's what you need to know — and when to seek help. Some couples seem to get pregnant simply by talking about it. For others, it takes plenty of patience and a bit of luck.

If you're hoping to join the ranks of other moms-to-be, start the old-fashioned way. Here's what you need to know — and when to seek help.

Baby-making basics

Conception is based on an intricate series of events.

Every month, hormones from your pituitary gland stimulate your ovaries to release an egg, or ovulate. This often happens around day 14 of the menstrual cycle, although the exact timing may vary among women or even from month to month.

Once the egg is released, it travels to the fallopian tube. If you want to conceive, now's the time. The egg has about 24 hours to unite with a sperm. Since sperm cells can survive in your reproductive tract for two to three days, it's best to have regular sex during the days leading up to ovulation.

If the egg is fertilized, it'll travel to the uterus two to four days later. There it'll attach to the uterine lining. You're pregnant! Your periods will stop as your body begins to support the embryo.

If the egg isn't fertilized, it'll break down and you'll have your next period as usual.

Understanding when you're most fertile

Learning how ovulation works is one thing. Determining when it's actually happening is something else. For many women, it's like hitting a moving target.

Keep an eye on the calendar: Use your day planner or another simple calendar to mark the day your period begins each month. Also track the number of days each period lasts.

If you have a consistent 28-day cycle, ovulation is likely to begin about 14 days after the day your last period began.

If your cycles are somewhat irregular, subtract 18 from the number of days in your shortest cycle. When your next period begins, count ahead this many days. This is a reasonable guess for your most fertile days.

- *Pros:* Calendar calculations can be done simply on paper. And they're free.
- *Cons:* Many factors may affect the exact timing of ovulation, including illness, stress and exercise. Counting days is often inaccurate, especially for women who have irregular cycles.

Watch for changes in cervical mucus: Just before ovulation, you'll notice an increase in clear, slippery vaginal secretions — if you check for it. These secretions typically resemble raw egg whites. After ovulation, when the odds of becoming pregnant are slim, the discharge will become cloudy and sticky or disappear entirely.

- *Pros:* Changes in vaginal secretions are often an accurate sign of impending fertility. Simple observation is all that's needed, particularly inside the vagina.
- *Cons:* Judging the texture or appearance of vaginal secretions can be somewhat subjective.

Track your basal body temperature: This is your body's temperature when you're at rest. Ovulation may cause a gradual rise in temperature or even a sudden jump — typically between 0.5 and 1.6 degrees Fahrenheit.

You'll be most fertile during the two to three days before your temperature rises. You can assume ovulation has occurred when the slightly higher temperature remains steady for three days or more.

Use an oral thermometer to monitor your basal body temperature. Try the digital variety or one specifically designed to measure basal body temperature. Simply take your temperature every morning before you get out of bed. Plot the readings on graph paper and look for a pattern to emerge.

- *Pros:* It's simple. The only cost is the thermometer. It's often most helpful to determine when you've ovulated and judge if the timing is consistent from month to month.
- *Cons:* The temperature change may be subtle, and the increase comes too late — after ovulation has already happened. It can be inconvenient to take your temperature

at the same time every day, especially if you have irregular sleeping hours.

Try an ovulation monitoring kit: Over-the-counter ovulation kits test your urine for the surge in hormones that takes place before ovulation. For the most accurate results, follow the instructions on the label to the letter.

- *Pros:* Ovulation kits can identify the most likely time of ovulation. They can even provide a signal before ovulation actually happens. They're available without a prescription in most pharmacies.

- *Cons:* Ovulation kits often lead to excessively targeted sex — and timing sex so precisely can invite being too late. The tests can also be expensive, often ranging from $20 to $50 each.

Maximizing fertility

When you're trying to conceive, consider these simple do's and don'ts.

Do:

- *Have sex regularly:* If you consistently have sex two or three times a week, you're almost certain to hit a fertile period at some point. For healthy couples who want to conceive, there's no such thing as too much sex. For many couples, this may be all it takes.

- *Have sex once a day near the time of ovulation:* Daily intercourse during the days leading up to ovulation may increase the odds of conception. Although your partner's sperm concentration will drop slightly each time you have sex, the reduction isn't an issue for healthy men.

- *Make healthy lifestyle choices:* Maintain a healthy weight, exercise regularly, eat healthfully and keep stress under control. The same good habits will serve you and your baby well during pregnancy.

- *Consider preconception planning:* Your doctor can assess your overall health and help you identify lifestyle changes that may improve your chances for a healthy pregnancy.

Preconception planning is especially helpful if you or your partner have any health issues.

- *Take your vitamins:* Folic acid (vitamin B-9) plays an essential role in a baby's development. Taking a prenatal vitamin or folic acid supplement beginning at least one month before conception through the first trimester of pregnancy can reduce the risk of spina bifida and other neural tube defects by up to 70 percent.

Don't:

- *Smoke:* Tobacco changes the cervical mucus, which may keep sperm from reaching the egg. Smoking may also increase the risk of miscarriage and deprive your developing baby of oxygen and nutrients. If you smoke, ask your doctor to help you quit before conception. For your family's sake, vow to quit for good.
- *Drink alcohol:* Alcohol is off limits if you're pregnant — or hope to be.
- *Take medication without your doctor's OK:* Certain medications— even those available without a prescription — can make it difficult to conceive. Others may not be safe once you're pregnant.

When to see your doctor

With frequent unprotected sex, most healthy couples conceive within six months. Ninety percent of healthy couples conceive within one year. Others need a bit of help.

If you're in your early 30s or younger and you and your partner are in good health, try it on your own for one year before consulting a doctor. You may want to seek help sooner if you're age 35 or older, your periods are more than 35 days apart, or you or your partner have known or suspected fertility issues.

Infertility affects men and women equally — and treatment is available. Depending on the source of the problem, your gynecologist, your partner's urologist or your family doctor may be able to help. In some cases, a fertility specialist may offer the best hope.

Preconception planning: Is your body ready for pregnancy?

There's more to pregnancy than maternity clothes and childbirth classes. A preconception appointment can help you make sure your body is up to the task. Here's what to expect. If you've decided you're ready to get pregnant, you may already be emotionally committed to parenthood. But is your body prepared for the task ahead?

To help ensure a healthy pregnancy, schedule a preconception appointment with your doctor. Be ready to discuss the following subjects.

Birth control

If you've been taking birth control pills, your doctor may recommend a pill-free break before trying to conceive. This will allow your reproductive system to go through several normal cycles — which will make it easier to more accurately determine when ovulation occurred and establish an expected due date.

During the pill-free break, you may want to use condoms or another barrier method of contraception.

Immunities

Infections such as chickenpox (varicella) and German measles (rubella) can cause serious disease for your unborn baby. If you aren't immune to these infections, your doctor may recommend being vaccinated at least one month before you try to conceive.

Chronic conditions

If you have a chronic medical condition — such as diabetes, asthma or high blood pressure — you'll want to make sure it's under control before you conceive. Your doctor will explain any special care you may need during pregnancy as well.

Family history

Sometimes family history — either your history or your partner's— increases the risk of having a child with certain conditions or birth defects. If genetic disorders are a concern, your doctor may refer you to a genetic counselor for a preconception assessment.

Medications and supplements

Tell your doctor about any medications, herbs or supplements you're taking. He or she may recommend changing doses or stopping them completely before you conceive.

This is also the time to begin taking a prenatal vitamin. Make sure it includes folic acid — a B vitamin that helps prevent serious birth defects in early pregnancy. Before conception and during pregnancy, you'll need 1 milligram (1,000 micrograms) of folic acid a day.

Age

After age 35, the risk of fertility problems, miscarriage and certain chromosomal disorders increases. Some pregnancy-related problems, such as high blood pressure and gestational diabetes, are more common in older mothers as well. Discuss these risks with your doctor and develop a plan for avoiding complications.

Previous pregnancies

Your doctor will ask about previous pregnancies. Be sure to mention any complications you may have had, such as high blood pressure, gestational diabetes, preterm labour, premature birth or birth defects. Share any concerns or fears you may have about another pregnancy. Your doctor will help you identify the best ways to boost the chances of a healthy pregnancy.

Lifestyle

Healthy lifestyle choices can help give your baby the best start. Your doctor will discuss eating healthy foods, exercising regularly and keeping stress under control. It's also important to avoid alcohol and recreational drugs. If you smoke, ask your doctor about resources to help you quit.

Your partner

If possible, have your partner attend the preconception visit with you. He can answer questions about his family medical history and risk factors for infections or birth defects. Your partner's health and lifestyle are important because they can affect you and your baby.

Pregnancy after 35: Healthy moms, healthy babies

Many women are delaying pregnancy well into their 30s and beyond— and delivering healthy babies. Take good care of yourself as you prepare for baby's arrival. If you're over 35 and hoping to get pregnant, you're in good company. Many women are delaying pregnancy well into their 30s and beyond — and delivering healthy babies. Take special care to give your baby the best start.

Understand the risks

The biological clock is a fact of life — but there's nothing magical about age 35. It's simply the age at which certain issues are recognised. For example:

It may take longer to get pregnant: You're born with all the eggs you'll ever have. As you reach your mid-30s, the eggs begin to decline in quality. After fertilization, an older egg is less likely to develop into a blastocyst — the ball of cells that implants into the uterus to begin a pregnancy.

Does this mean you can't get pregnant? No. Many older women successfully conceive, but it may take a bit longer. If you're over 35 and have been unable to conceive for six to nine months, you may want to consult your health care provider for advice.

You're more likely to have a multiple pregnancy: Age-related hormonal changes may cause you to release more than one egg at a time, which boosts the odds of conceiving nonidentical (fraternal) twins.

Because of their decreased fertility, older women are also more likely to use assisted reproductive technologies — such as in vitro fertilization— to conceive. Since these procedures typically involve implanting more than one fertilized egg in the uterus, they're more likely to result in twins or other multiples.

The risk of miscarriage is higher: Sadly, the risk of miscarriage increases as you get older. Here's the breakdown:

- Before age 35 — 15 percent risk
- Ages 35 to 39 — 20 to 25 percent risk
- Ages 40 to 42 — 35 percent risk
- After age 42 — 50 percent risk

You're more likely to develop gestational diabetes: This type of diabetes occurs only during pregnancy. Tight control of blood sugar through diet, exercise and other lifestyle measures is essential to prevent complications. Sometimes, medication is needed as well. Your treatment plan may include frequent prenatal checkups and regular blood sugar testing at home.

You may need a Caesarean section: Many factors may be at play here. For example:

- Older mothers have a higher risk of pregnancy-related complications, such as high blood pressure and gestational diabetes. These problems can lead to Caesarean delivery.
- There's a greater chance that your cervix will be slow to dilate, which also may lead to a C-section.
- If your baby is too big or you've gained too much weight — common issues for older mothers — vaginal delivery may be difficult.
- Babies of older mothers are more likely to be in a position that complicates vaginal delivery, such as rump-first or feet-first (breech).
- Placenta previa — a condition in which the placenta either partially or completely covers the cervix — may lead to a C-section.
- C-sections are often recommended for multiple births.

The risk of chromosome abnormalities is higher: Babies born to older mothers have a higher risk of various chromosome problems, such as Down syndrome. At age 30, the risk of Down syndrome is about one in 1,000 live births. At age 35, it's about one in 400. By age 40, the risk is about one in 100.

Make healthy choices

Taking good care of yourself is the best way to take care of your baby. Pay special attention to the basics.

Make a preconception appointment: Meet with your health care provider before you conceive to make sure your body is prepared for the task ahead. He or she will assess your overall health and discuss lifestyle changes that may improve your chances for a healthy pregnancy and baby.

The preconception appointment is a great time to address any concerns you may have about fertility or pregnancy at your age. Ask the best ways to boost the odds of conception — and the options if you have trouble conceiving.

Seek regular prenatal care: During pregnancy, regular prenatal visits can help your health care provider monitor your health and your baby's health. Mention any signs or symptoms that concern you, even if they seem silly or unimportant. Talking to your health care provider is likely to put your mind at ease.

Eat healthfully: During pregnancy, you'll need more folic acid, calcium, iron, protein and other essential nutrients. If you're already eating healthfully, keep it up. A daily prenatal vitamin — ideally starting before conception — can help fill any gaps.

Gain weight wisely: Gaining the right amount of weight can support your baby's health — and make it easier to shed the extra pounds after delivery. Work with your health care provider to determine what's right for you. Here are the general guidelines:

Pre-pregnancy weight	*Recommended weight gain*
Underweight	28 to 40 pounds
Normal weight	25 to 35 pounds
Overweight	15 to 25 pounds
Obese	At least 15 pounds

If you're carrying twins or triplets, you'll need to gain more weight— often 35 to 45 pounds.

Stay physically active: Unless your health care provider prescribes bed rest, pregnancy can be a great time to get active. Exercise can help ease or even prevent discomfort, boost your energy level and improve your overall health. Perhaps best of all, it can help you prepare for labour and childbirth by increasing your stamina and muscle strength.

Get your health care provider's OK before starting or continuing an exercise programme — especially if you have a medical condition or history of preterm labour.

Avoid risky substances: Alcohol, tobacco and recreational drugs are off-limits during pregnancy. Even moderate or minimal alcohol use can harm your developing baby. Smoking increases the risk of preterm birth, problems with the placenta and certain birth defects. Any drugs you take can pass from you to your baby, sometimes with devastating effects. Even prescription and over-the-counter medications deserve caution. Clear any medications or supplements with your health care provider ahead of time.

Learn about prenatal testing for chromosomal abnormalities: Diagnostic tests such as chorionic villus sampling and genetic amniocentesis can provide information about your baby's chromosomes, but at a small risk of losing the pregnancy. Your health care provider can help you weigh this risk against the value you place in having the information. Typically, prenatal tests simply confirm that a baby is healthy. But it's important to be prepared for other possibilities. Trust your health care provider to help you make decisions consistent with your own values.

Look toward the future

The choices you make now — even before conception — can have a lasting effect on your baby. Think of pregnancy as an opportunity to nurture your baby and prepare for the exciting changes ahead.

Pregnancy: When you have a chronic health condition

Pregnancy becomes more complicated when you have a chronic health condition. Learn the importance of preconception planning and regular prenatal care.

Are you ready to have a baby? It's an important question for any woman — but the decision may be more complicated if you have a chronic health condition. Work with your health care provider to make the best choices for you and your baby.

Start with a preconception appointment

A preconception appointment can help you make sure your body is prepared for the challenge of pregnancy. Your health care provider will evaluate how well you're managing your condition and explain any special care you may need during pregnancy.

It's also the time to ask questions.

- *Will it be tough to conceive?* Some chronic conditions — or their treatments — may affect your ability to get pregnant. For example, women who have epilepsy may have menstrual cycle irregularities that interfere with fertility. Women who have hypothyroidism may have difficulty becoming pregnant as well.

- *How will pregnancy affect my condition?* Every woman reacts differently to pregnancy. Sometimes signs and symptoms of a chronic condition remain the same or even improve during pregnancy — particularly for autoimmune conditions such as rheumatoid arthritis. However, pregnancy also aggravates some chronic conditions. Make sure you're prepared for the toll pregnancy may take on your physical and emotional health.

- *What are the risks?* Some chronic conditions pose potentially serious risks for you or your baby — particularly if they're managed poorly. For example, uncontrolled asthma may decrease your baby's oxygen supply. High blood pressure may cause problems with the placenta or your baby's growth. Diabetes may increase your baby's birth weight. Sometimes birth defects are a concern.

- *How should I prepare for pregnancy?* To give your baby the best start, make sure your condition is under control before you conceive. Healthy lifestyle choices are essential as well. Lose excess weight. Eat healthfully. Take prenatal vitamins, including folic acid. Exercise regularly. Keep stress under control. Avoid smoking, alcohol and recreational drugs.

- *Will my treatment change during pregnancy?* Some treatment plans can continue throughout pregnancy. Others may need to be adjusted. Your health care provider will tailor a treatment plan based on your individual needs.

- *What about medication?* Any medication you take during pregnancy may affect your baby. But often the benefits outweigh the risks. Depending on the circumstances, your health care provider may switch you to a similar drug that's safer during pregnancy or prescribe medication only during certain stages of your pregnancy.

- *How can I boost the odds of having a healthy baby?* Women who have chronic conditions deliver healthy babies every day. Follow your health care provider's recommendations for taking care of yourself and your baby.

- *Will I be able to breast-feed my baby?* Breast-feeding is encouraged for many women with chronic conditions — even those who take medication. Before you begin breast-feeding, talk with your health care provider about any adjustments you may need to make to your treatment plan.

Seek regular prenatal care

If you decide to become pregnant, your health care provider will closely monitor you throughout your pregnancy. Consistent visits will help him or her keep an eye on your underlying condition and detect any problems quickly. If you're taking medication, you may need adjustments as your pregnancy progresses.

Your baby's health will be closely monitored as well. Frequent ultrasounds may be used to track your baby's growth and development. Depending on the circumstances, your health care provider may recommend other prenatal tests, such as amniocentesis or chorionic villus sampling. What you learn may help you understand the odds and make important decisions.

Focus on a healthy baby

If your chronic condition poses risks for you or your baby, nine months may seem like an impossibly long time to wonder — and worry— about your pregnancy. Share your concerns with your health care provider. Seek support from your partner, loved ones and friends. Find local support groups or online chat rooms for women in similar situations. Take comfort in the thought that you're doing everything you can to promote a healthy pregnancy.

┌─────┐
│ **7** │
└─────┘

Pregnancy Complications

COMPLICATIONS

Each year, ill health as a result of pregnancy is experienced (sometimes permanently) by more than 20 million women around the world. In 2016, complications of pregnancy resulted in 230,600 deaths down from 377,000 deaths in 1990. Common causes include bleeding (72,000), infections (20,000), hypertensive diseases of pregnancy (32,000), obstructed labor (10,000), and pregnancy with abortive outcome (20,000), which includes miscarriage, abortion, and ectopic pregnancy.

The following are some examples of pregnancy complications:
- Pregnancy induced hypertension
- Anemia
- Postpartum depression
- Postpartum psychosis
- Thromboembolic disorders, with an increased risk due to hypercoagulability in pregnancy. These are the leading cause of death in pregnant women in the US.
- Pruritic urticarial papules and plaques of pregnancy (PUPPP), a skin disease that develops around the 32nd week. Signs are red plaques, papules, and itchiness around the belly button that then spreads all over the body except for the inside of hands and face.
- Ectopic pregnancy, including abdominal pregnancy, implantation of the embryo outside the uterus

- Hyperemesis gravidarum, excessive nausea and vomiting that is more severe than normal morning sickness.
- Pulmonary embolism, a blood clot that forms in the legs and migrates to the lungs.
- Acute fatty liver of pregnancy is a rare complication thought to be brought about by a disruption in the metabolism of fatty acids by mitochondria.

There is also an increased susceptibility and severity of certain infections in pregnancy.

GESTATIONAL DIABETES

Gestational diabetes is a type of diabetes that occurs only during pregnancy. Like other forms of diabetes, gestational diabetes affects the way your body uses blood sugar (glucose) — your body's main source of fuel. As a result, your blood sugar level is too high.

If untreated or uncontrolled, gestational diabetes can result in a variety of health problems for you and your baby.

If you have gestational diabetes, you and your doctor will devise a plan to keep your blood sugar levels within a normal range. The good news is that controlling your blood sugar can help ensure a healthy pregnancy for you and a healthy start for your baby.

Signs and symptoms: Most women don't experience any signs or symptoms of gestational diabetes. When they do occur, signs and symptoms may include:

- Excessive thirst
- Increased urination

Causes: During digestion, your body breaks carbohydrates into simple sugar molecules that it can eventually use for energy. One of these sugar molecules is glucose, the main energy source for your body. Glucose is absorbed directly into your bloodstream after you eat, but it can't enter your cells without the help of insulin.

Your pancreas — a gland located just behind your stomach — produces insulin continuously. The insulin "escorts" sugar into your cells, providing your body with energy while maintaining a normal level of sugar in your blood.

Your liver also plays a key role in maintaining a normal blood sugar level. If you have more glucose than your cells need for energy, your body can remove that excess from your bloodstream and store it in your liver as glycogen. Then, when you run low on glucose — for example, if you haven't eaten for a while — your body can tap into that stored glucose and release it into your bloodstream.

The amount of glucose in your blood fluctuates in response to a number of factors, including the food you eat, exercise, stress and infections. Yet the complex relationship among insulin, glucose and your liver ensures that your blood sugar stays within set limits.

During pregnancy, your placenta — the organ that supplies your baby with nutrients through the umbilical cord — produces hormones that prevent insulin from doing its job. These hormones, which include estrogen, cortisol and human placental lactogen, are vital to preserving your pregnancy. Yet they also make your cells more resistant to insulin.

As your placenta grows larger in the second and third trimesters, it secretes even more of these hormones, further increasing insulin resistance. Normally, your pancreas responds by producing enough extra insulin to overcome this resistance. But you may need up to three times as much insulin as normal, and sometimes your pancreas simply can't keep up. When this happens, too little glucose gets into your cells and too much stays in your blood. This is gestational diabetes. It usually occurs about the 20th to 24th week of pregnancy and can be measured by the 24th to 28th week of pregnancy. After your baby is born and placental hormones disappear from your bloodstream, your blood sugar levels should quickly return to normal.

Risk factors: Any woman can develop gestational diabetes, but some women are at greater risk than are others. These factors increase your risk:

- *Age:* Women older than age 25 are more likely to develop gestational diabetes.

- *Family or personal history:* Your chance of developing gestational diabetes increases if a close family member, such as a parent or sibling, has type 2 diabetes. You're also more likely to have gestational diabetes if you've had it in a previous pregnancy.
- *Weight:* Being overweight before pregnancy makes it more likely that you'll develop gestational diabetes. However, gaining weight during your pregnancy doesn't cause gestational diabetes.
- *Race:* For reasons that aren't clear, women of some races are more likely to develop gestational diabetes than are others. You're at increased risk if you're black, Hispanic or American Indian.
- *Previous complicated pregnancy:* If you've had an unexplained stillbirth or a baby who weighed more than 9 pounds, you may be screened more closely for gestational diabetes the next time you become pregnant.

Many women who develop gestational diabetes have no known risk factors.

When to seek medical advice?: Your health care provider will address gestational diabetes as part of your regular prenatal care. If you develop gestational diabetes, see your health care provider for regular checkups. How often you see your provider depends on the severity of your diabetes and whether you have any other complications. Office visits with your health care provider are especially important during the final three months of your pregnancy, when he or she will carefully monitor your blood sugar levels.

In addition, your health care provider may refer you to other health professionals who specialise in the management of diabetes, such as an endocrinologist, a registered dietitian or a diabetes educator. They can help you learn to manage your blood sugar during your pregnancy. In some cases, your health care provider may refer you to — or consult with— a doctor who specialises in high-risk pregnancies.

To make sure that your glucose level has returned to normal after your baby is born, you'll have your blood sugar checked often after delivery and again in six weeks. Once you've had gestational diabetes, continue to have your blood sugar tested at least once a year. And continue healthy lifestyle habits to lessen your chances of developing type 2 diabetes.

Screening and diagnosis: In some places, screening for gestational diabetes is a routine part of prenatal care for all women. Until recently, though, there was no scientific proof that screening resulted in fewer childbirth complications and healthier babies. In a 2005 study, researchers screened pregnant women for gestational diabetes and randomly assigned those with gestational diabetes to receive aggressive or routine treatment. The outcome — healthier babies and fewer childbirth complications for women who received aggressive treatment — demonstrated the wisdom of screening all mothers.

To screen for gestational diabetes, most doctors recommend a glucose challenge test. This test is usually done between 24 and 28 weeks of pregnancy, because the condition usually can't be detected until then. However, if your doctor thinks you're especially at risk, the test may be performed earlier.

If you're younger than 25 and have no other risk factors for gestational diabetes, there is some debate about whether you should undergo the test. Some doctors argue that younger women don't need this test. Others say that screening all pregnant women — no matter their age — is the best way to catch all cases of the disease.

What to expect from the test?: When you arrive for a glucose challenge test, you'll be asked to drink a glucose solution that tastes like extra-sweet soda pop. Then you're in for a one-hour wait, before a blood sample is drawn from a vein in your arm to determine your blood sugar level. The glucose drink may make you feel nauseous or dizzy. But the syrupy solution — and the wait — are necessary to tell how efficiently your body processes sugar.

A blood sugar level below 140 milligrams per deciliter (mg/dL) is usually considered normal on a glucose challenge test. Having a blood sugar level above 140 mg/dL doesn't necessarily mean you have gestational diabetes. To confirm the diagnosis, you'll need a second test. For the follow-up test, you'll be asked to fast overnight. You're then given another sweet solution to drink — this one containing a higher concentration of glucose — and your blood sugar levels are checked every hour for a period of three hours. Having at least two instances of abnormally high blood sugar levels confirms the diagnosis of gestational diabetes.

Why these tests?: Some women wonder why it's necessary to undergo these screening tests in addition to routine urine samples. A urine sample isn't a reliable indicator of gestational diabetes because the amount of sugar in your urine can vary throughout the day and as a result of what you eat. Screening tests are a much better way to identify women with gestational diabetes.

Complications: Some women worry that having gestational diabetes will cause birth defects. Fortunately, this usually isn't the case. In general, birth defects originate during the first three months of pregnancy, while gestational diabetes generally doesn't develop until the second or third trimester. This means your blood sugar levels are normal during the first critical months.

Most women with gestational diabetes go on to deliver healthy babies. However, untreated or uncontrolled blood sugar levels can cause problems for you and your baby.

Complications that may affect your baby: Consistently keeping your blood sugar levels within a normal range can reduce these possible complications:

- *Macrosomia:* Extra glucose can cross the placenta and end up in your baby's blood. When that happens, your baby's pancreas makes extra insulin to process the extra glucose, and this can cause your baby to grow too large (macrosomia). For a full-term pregnancy, this means a birth weight of 4,500 grams (9 pounds, 14 ounces) or more. Very large babies may have difficulty during delivery and are more likely to sustain birth injuries or be born by Caesarean delivery.

- *Shoulder dystocia:* If you have a very large baby, your baby's shoulders may be too big to move through the birth canal. This results in a potentially life-threatening obstetrical emergency, known as shoulder dystocia. In most cases, doctors can perform maneuvers to free the baby, but injuries may occur under the best of care. This is a rare but very serious complication of gestational diabetes.

- *Hypoglycemia:* Sometimes babies of mothers with gestational diabetes develop low blood sugar (hypoglycemia) shortly after birth. That's because they're accustomed to receiving large amounts of blood sugar from their mothers, and their own insulin production is high. These infants should have their blood sugar levels checked regularly after delivery. Treating this problem involves feeding right away. Your baby may even need a glucose solution through an intravenous line to prevent low blood sugar.

- *Respiratory distress syndrome:* Babies born prematurely to mothers with gestational diabetes are more likely to develop respiratory distress syndrome, a condition that makes breathing difficult. It's caused by a lack of certain substances in the lungs that help prevent the lungs from collapsing every time the baby takes a breath. Babies with respiratory distress syndrome may need help breathing until their lungs become stronger.

- *Jaundice:* This yellowish discoloration of the skin and the whites of the eyes is another potential complication. Newborn jaundice may begin during the second or third day of life, but sometimes isn't evident until around a week after birth. Jaundice itself isn't a disease. In most cases it occurs because a baby's liver isn't mature enough to break down a substance called bilirubin, which normally forms when the body recycles old or damaged red blood cells. Although jaundice usually isn't a cause for concern, it should be carefully monitored by your doctor.

- *Stillbirth or death:* If gestational diabetes goes undetected, a baby has an increased risk of stillbirth or death as a newborn.

Complications that may affect you: If you have gestational diabetes, you may be at risk of these complications:

- *Preeclampsia:* This condition is primarily characterised by a significant increase in blood pressure. Left untreated, it can lead to serious, even deadly complications for the mother and fetus. Having gestational diabetes puts you at higher risk of developing this condition, so you'll want to discuss it with your doctor.

- *Operative delivery:* Gestational diabetes isn't a reason to schedule a Caesarean delivery. But your doctor may recommend one if your baby has macrosomia.

- *Gestational diabetes in another pregnancy:* Once you've had gestational diabetes in one pregnancy, you're more likely to have it again with the next pregnancy.

- *Type 2 diabetes:* Women who have gestational diabetes are more likely to develop type 2 diabetes — a type of diabetes that's present all the time, not just during pregnancy — as they get older. Many cases of diabetes can be prevented with a healthy diet and regular exercise.

Treatment: Controlling your blood sugar is essential to keeping your baby healthy and avoiding complications during delivery. Most women with gestational diabetes are able to control their blood sugar with diet and exercise, but some may need medication in addition to lifestyle changes. In either case, monitoring your blood sugar is a key part of your treatment programme because it tells you whether your blood sugar is staying within a normal range.

The most recent data support aggressively treating all pregnant women with gestational diabetes. Evidence favoring aggressive treatment comes from the same 2005 study that proved the benefit of screening all pregnant women for gestational diabetes. Researchers compared pregnancy outcomes in two groups of women with gestational diabetes. One group received aggressive treatment — dietary advice, frequent blood glucose monitoring and insulin injections for elevated blood glucose levels. Another goal of aggressive treatment was to maintain tight control of blood glucose. The blood glucose goals for this group were 63 to 99 milligrams of glucose per deciliter (mg/dL) for fasting blood sugar and 126 mg/dL or lower two hours after meals. The other group received routine care, which may or may not have included insulin.

The women who received aggressive treatment and maintained tighter glucose control developed significantly fewer childbirth problems than did the women who had routine care. Aggressive treatment was particularly effective in reducing the types of problems caused by having unusually large babies, as women with high blood glucose during pregnancy often do.

In addition, the group that received aggressive treatment reported lower rates of depression and scored higher on health-related quality of life three months after giving birth than did the group receiving routine care. It isn't clear, however, why these particular benefits occurred.

Monitoring your blood sugar: If you've just learned that you have diabetes, monitoring your blood sugar may sound inconvenient and difficult. But once you learn how it's done, you'll likely grow more comfortable with the procedure.

To test your blood sugar, you draw a drop of blood from your finger using a small needle (lancet), then place the blood on a test strip inserted into a blood glucose meter — a small, computerised device that measures and displays your blood sugar level.

Your blood sugar fluctuates throughout the day. What and how much you eat and even the time of day also can have an effect. For that reason, your doctor may ask you to check your blood sugar four to five times a day. Your goal is to make sure you're keeping your blood sugar levels within a healthy range.

Your doctor will also monitor your blood sugar during labour. If your blood sugar levels rise, your baby's blood sugar will rise, too. This can cause your baby to have high levels of insulin, which may lead to low blood sugar right after birth.

Eating a healthy diet: A healthy diet is important for every pregnant woman, but it's even more important if you have gestational diabetes. Eating the right kind and amount of food is one of the best ways to control your blood sugar levels.

In general, you'll need more fruits, vegetables and whole grains — foods that are high in nutrition and low in fat and calories — and fewer animal products and sweets. Even so, no one diet is right for every woman. If you have gestational diabetes, work with a registered dietitian or counselor who can help you put together an individual meal plan based on your blood sugar level, height, weight, exercise habits and food preferences.

Getting regular exercise: In general, the more active you are, the lower your blood sugar. Physical activity causes sugar to be transported to your cells where it's used for energy, lowering the levels in your blood. Exercise also reduces blood sugar by increasing your sensitivity to insulin: Your body requires less insulin to transport glucose into your cells.

In addition, regular exercise can help prevent some of the discomforts of pregnancy, such as back pain, muscle cramps, swelling, constipation and difficulty sleeping. It can also help prepare you for labour and delivery. The increased muscle strength and endurance you develop reduce stress on your ligaments and joints during delivery, help you during labour, and shorten your recovery time.

Your doctor will discuss exercise as a part of the treatment for gestational diabetes. Once you understand the ground rules, take some time to think about which activities you enjoy. Walking, cycling and swimming are good ways to get a safe aerobic workout. Ordinary activities such as housework and gardening also can lower your blood sugar.

Aim for moderate aerobic exercise on most days. If you haven't been active for a while, start slowly and build up gradually. For best results, combine aerobic activity with stretching and strength-training exercises. Exercising at the same time every day, varying your fitness routine and working out with other pregnant women can help you stay motivated.

Taking medications: Sometimes diet and exercise may not be enough. In that case, you may need to take daily medication to help lower your blood sugar to safe levels.

Until recently, insulin was the only option for women with gestational diabetes because it doesn't cross the placental barrier. But the oral anti-diabetes drug, glyburide, also may be safe and effective in controlling blood sugar in gestational diabetes. Doctors in Europe use metformin to treat gestational diabetes, and this medication is being studied in the United States.

Monitoring your baby: Your obstetrician will likely recommend close monitoring of your baby's growth — usually using ultrasound. This test combines high-frequency sound waves and computer processing to generate pictures of the inside of your uterus. Although ultrasound can give a good idea of your baby's size, it tends to be less accurate as your baby gets bigger.

If you need medications to control your gestational diabetes, your obstetrician may also recommend a nonstress test (NST) or biophysical profile to make sure your baby is getting enough oxygen and nourishment, especially as you approach your due date. A nonstress test is just that— a noninvasive test that causes no stress to your baby. In fact, it shouldn't be stressful for you either. NST usually takes less than 30 minutes and requires no hospitalization. It's a simple procedure that checks how often your baby moves and how much his or her heart rate increases with movement. A biophysical profile combines an ultrasound with NST to provide more information about your baby's breathing, tone, movement and the volume of amniotic fluid in your uterus.

In most cases, your doctor will try to prevent your pregnancy from going longer than 40 weeks because being overdue may increase the risk of complications. Although most women with gestational diabetes deliver happy, healthy babies, labour with gestational diabetes isn't routine, and Caesarean delivery is necessary in some cases. However, gestational diabetes doesn't affect your ability to breast-feed or care for your new baby.

Coping skills: It's not easy to live with a condition that can affect the health of your unborn child. Although most of the complications of gestational diabetes can be prevented with diet and exercise, it can be stressful to regularly monitor your blood sugar and follow a specific diet and exercise plan.

Besides, worrying about your baby can make it harder to take care of yourself and manage your condition. You may actually find yourself eating all of the wrong foods or forgetting to exercise. Prolonged stress can even cause your blood sugar levels to rise.

You'll probably feel better if you learn as much as you can about your condition. In addition to talking to your doctor and a diabetes educator or dietitian, look for information in books or on the Internet. Ask your doctor to put you in touch with other women who have the same disorder.

And remember: The very steps you're taking to control your blood sugar — such as eating a healthy diet and getting regular exercise — can help relieve stress and nourish your baby. These activities may also help prevent you from developing type 2 diabetes in the future. That makes exercise and good nutrition your most powerful tools for a healthy life as well as for a healthy pregnancy.

Placenta previa

At the very beginning of pregnancy, the placenta begins to form. This circular, flat organ is responsible for providing oxygen and nutrients to your growing baby and removing waste products from your baby's blood. It attaches to the wall of your uterus and your baby's umbilical cord, forming a vital connection between you and your baby.

Early in pregnancy, the placenta may implant in the lower part of your uterus. However, as your uterus grows, the placenta usually moves up and away from the opening of your uterus, called your cervix. If it doesn't, it's called placenta previa.

This condition occurs in about one in 200 pregnancies, and it can be dangerous for both you and your baby. When the placenta covers the opening to your cervix, the placenta will detach from that part of your uterus as your cervix begins to thin and dilate in preparation for labour. This can cause severe vaginal bleeding.

In fact, most women with placenta previa experience moderate to heavy bleeding in the second half of pregnancy. This can be scary, but the bleeding will alert your health care provider to the condition — if it wasn't already detected by ultrasound. Then you can make plans to treat it.

Signs and symptoms: Painless, bright red vaginal bleeding in the second half of pregnancy is the main sign of placenta previa. This bleeding usually occurs near the end of the second trimester or the beginning of the third. The amount of bleeding may range from light to heavy. And it may stop, but it nearly always recurs days or weeks later.

Some women with placenta previa experience contractions with bleeding. In addition, some women have light bleeding or spotting during the first trimester or early second trimester. Today, most cases of placenta previa are discovered by a routine ultrasound, done as part of your prenatal care, before any bleeding takes place.

Types of placenta previa: There are three types of placenta previa, but they all cause the same general signs and symptoms. An ultrasound is necessary to tell which form of the condition you have:

- *Total placenta previa:* In total placenta previa, the placenta completely covers the cervical opening.
- *Partial placenta previa:* In partial placenta previa, the placenta partly covers the cervical opening.
- *Marginal placenta previa:* In marginal placenta previa, the edge of the placenta is at the margin of the cervical opening. This form of placenta previa may not cause much bleeding, and it may be possible for your baby to make its way into the birth canal without any difficulty.

"Low-lying placenta" is another term related to placenta previa. This term is usually used to describe a placenta that lies low in the uterus but isn't quite close enough to the cervical opening to qualify as marginal placenta previa. This condition usually doesn't require treatment during pregnancy, but it may cause bleeding after delivery.

Causes: Placenta previa occurs when the embryo implants in the lower part of the uterus and then grows to cover the exit.

Doctors and researchers don't understand why this happens. They hypothesise that the condition may be related to:
- Scars in the lining of the uterus (endometrium)
- A large placenta, such as in multiple pregnancy
- An abnormally shaped uterus

Risk factors: The most significant risk factor for placenta previa is a previous Caesarean birth. However, other factors may also increase your risk of developing the condition:
- Having had placenta previa before
- Having had other children
- Being age 35 and older
- Smoking
- Carrying twins, triplets or more

Previous uterine surgeries, such as myomectomy to remove uterine fibroids or dilation and curettage (D and C), in which the lining of the uterus is scraped for medical reasons, also seem to increase the risk of placenta previa.

When to seek medical advice?: If you're pregnant, seek regular prenatal care. If you experience any vaginal bleeding during your second or third trimester, call your health care provider right away. Your health care provider will want to perform an ultrasound to determine if you have placenta previa or some other condition.

If you have already been diagnosed with placenta previa, make sure that any health care provider you see during pregnancy is aware of the condition. This news will change the care you receive.

For example, women with placenta previa usually don't have digital vaginal exams, because even the gentlest vaginal exam can trigger severe bleeding. For the same reason, you'll probably be advised to avoid sexual intercourse, exercise and certain medications. Make sure to discuss do's and don'ts with your doctor

Screening and diagnosis: Placenta previa is discovered by ultrasound, during a routine prenatal appointment or after an episode of vaginal bleeding. The condition is almost always detected before a woman or her baby is in significant danger.

But this is just another reason to get regular prenatal exams.

Diagnosis before 20 weeks of pregnancy: You may be told that you have a low-lying placenta or placenta previa before 20 weeks of pregnancy, based on the results of a routine ultrasound. This is fairly common. Up to 15 percent of pregnant women show some evidence of a low-lying placenta or placenta previa during their midpregnancy ultrasound. More than 90 percent of these cases spontaneously resolve before delivery, as the uterus grows and the placenta migrates away from the opening of the uterus.

However, your health care provider will monitor you closely to make sure that's the case. You may need extra ultrasounds to track the position of your placenta. The longer the placenta previa persists, the more likely it will be present at delivery.

Diagnosis after 20 weeks of pregnancy: Your health care provider may detect placenta previa late in pregnancy during an ultrasound for some unrelated reason. However, at this stage of pregnancy, vaginal bleeding is typically the tip-off.

If you experience vaginal bleeding in the second or third trimester, you'll need to go to your doctor's office or the hospital to determine the cause of the bleeding. Placenta previa is one of the first things your health care provider will look for. In most cases, an abdominal ultrasound can identify the location of your placenta, so your health care provider can quickly confirm or rule out this condition. But a definitive diagnosis may require a combination of abdominal ultrasound and transvaginal ultrasound— which requires a wand-like device placed inside your vagina.

If your health care provider suspects that you may have placenta previa, he or she won't do a vaginal exam, because it can trigger heavy bleeding. But you may undergo additional ultrasounds or magnetic resonance imaging (MRI) to detect the exact location of your placenta before delivery. These tests don't use radiation, like an X-ray, so there is no harm to your baby. If you have placenta previa, you may also be hooked up to monitors that check your baby's well-being.

Complications: If you have placenta previa, your doctor will monitor you and your baby carefully to reduce your risk of these serious complications:

- *Massive bleeding (hemorrhage):* One of the biggest concerns with placenta previa is the risk of severe vaginal bleeding, which can be heavy enough to cause maternal shock or even death.
- *Premature birth:* Placenta previa can lead to premature birth. Some women with severe bleeding actually need an emergency Caesarean birth sometime in the third trimester.
- *Placenta accreta:* In this condition, the placenta implants too deeply and firmly into the uterine wall, making it difficult for the placenta to spontaneously detach from the uterus after delivery. This can result in severe bleeding and the need for the surgical removal of the uterus (hysterectomy). This condition is rare, but it typically affects women with placenta previa or women who have had a previous Caesarean birth or some other uterine surgery.

Related conditions: These conditions are often grouped with placenta previa because they can cause vaginal bleeding in the late second or third trimesters. If you have vaginal bleeding late in your pregnancy, your health care provider will consider all three conditions before making a diagnosis.

- *Placental abruption:* Sometimes called abruptio placentae, this rare condition occurs when the placenta begins to separate from the inner wall of the uterus before birth. It can deprive the baby of oxygen and nutrients and cause heavy bleeding within the uterus that may be dangerous for the mother and her baby. Placental abruption can be a complication of placenta previa, but most abruptions happen in women without placenta previa.
- *Vasa previa:* In this rare condition, the umbilical cord develops in an abnormal place instead of in the center of the placenta, which allows the fetus's blood vessels to cross the cervix. This can result in rupture of the blood vessels, which causes life-threatening bleeding in the baby.

Treatment: In general, treatment for placenta previa may include blood transfusions, bed rest and Caesarean delivery. But the details of your treatment depend on a range of factors, including:

- The amount of vaginal bleeding
- Whether the bleeding has stopped
- The gestational age of your baby
- Your health
- Your baby's health
- The position of the placenta and the baby

For marginal placenta previa or other forms with little or no bleeding: If you have marginal placenta previa that was diagnosed during a routine ultrasound or another form of placenta previa but little or no bleeding, you may be allowed to rest at home, rather than being admitted to the hospital. But your doctor will want to see you regularly, to monitor your blood levels, your baby's development and the position of your placenta.

The rules for bed rest depend on your individual situation. You may need to lie in bed, only sitting and standing when necessary. Or you may be advised to sit on the couch or in bed and to limit your activities. Either way, you'll need to avoid sexual intercourse, exercise and vaginal exams, which can trigger bleeding. You'll also want to avoid nonsteroidal anti-inflammatory drugs (NSAIDs) such as aspirin and ibuprofen, unless your doctor recommends them, because these medications may contribute to bleeding. And you'll need to seek emergency medical attention if vaginal bleeding starts.

If your placenta doesn't cover the opening of your uterus, you may be allowed to attempt a vaginal delivery. But you'll be monitored closely, and you may need a Caesarean birth if there is heavy vaginal bleeding.

For severe bleeding: After an initial bleeding episode, women with placenta previa are often kept in the hospital, where a Caesarean birth is planned for as soon as the baby can be safely delivered. Ideally, your doctor will try to manage your condition until you've reached 36 weeks of pregnancy. In more severe cases, it may not be possible to wait, and you may need to undergo Caesarean birth earlier.

If bleeding is severe, you may need a blood transfusion to replace lost blood. If bleeding occurs before the last few weeks of your pregnancy, you may also need medications to prevent premature labour, as well as corticosteroids. These potent medications can help make your baby's lungs more mature in as little as 48 hours. Underdeveloped lungs are one of the biggest problems facing premature infants, so corticosteroids can be an important step in helping an immature baby prepare for life outside of the uterus.

For bleeding that won't stop: If bleeding starts and can't be controlled, an emergency Caesarean birth is necessary for the sake of the mother and baby — even if the baby is premature. You may also undergo urgent Caesarean birth if monitors show a problem with your baby's heart rate.

Coping skills: Pregnancy is supposed to be a time of awe and anticipation. Nine months of watching your belly grow and waiting to meet the little one inside. Nine months for picking out the softest quilt, the safest crib and the right rocking chair. A condition that could cause excessive bleeding before or during delivery isn't part of any mother's vision of the perfect pregnancy. Yet most women with placenta previa go on to deliver a happy, healthy baby — which is far better than a perfect pregnancy.

Still, if you're diagnosed with placenta previa, you're sure to be scared, anxious and worried about how your condition will affect your baby. Some of these strategies may help:

- *Learn about placenta previa:* Gathering information about your condition may help you feel less scared. Talk to your doctor, do some research on your own and ask your doctor to put you in touch with other women who have had placenta previa.
- *Learn about Caesarean birth:* Most women with placenta previa will have a Caesarean birth, so it's smart to talk about this procedure in advance. Take time to ask your

doctor every question that comes to mind. If you're feeling disappointed that you won't deliver vaginally, talk about your feelings and ask about ways to make your birth as "natural" as possible, such as having your partner hold the baby close to you right away.

- *Make the best of bed rest:* If you're put on bed rest, fill your days by planning for your baby's arrival. Read about newborn care or purchase newborn necessities, either online or from catalogs. Or use your time to balance your checkbook, organise old photo albums or catch up on thank-you notes.

- *Take care of yourself:* Aside from following your treatment plan, you can't do anything to help your condition except to wait. But you can take steps to take care of yourself. Surround yourself with things that bring you comfort, such as prayer, a good book or a favorite pair of pajamas. Ask your mom to bring over her famous apple pie, or ask your best friends to stop by for a visit. Your partner, friends and family are likely looking for ways to help, so they'll be glad for a concrete suggestion.

PLACENTAL ABRUPTION

The placenta is a structure that develops in the uterus during pregnancy to nourish the growing baby. If the placenta separates from the inner wall of the uterus before delivery, it's known as placental abruption. This rare— but serious — complication of pregnancy requires immediate medical attention.

With placental abruption, the uterus bleeds from the site where the placenta was attached. The blood typically passes through the cervix and out the vagina. Sometimes, however, the blood remains trapped behind the placenta. Left untreated, placental abruption puts both mother and baby in jeopardy.

Placental abruption is most common in the third trimester, but it can begin any time after 20 weeks of pregnancy. With close monitoring and delivery at the appropriate time, the outlook is promising.

Signs and symptoms: In the early stages of placental abruption, you may not have any signs or symptoms.

Bleeding from the vagina is often the first sign. The amount of bleeding can vary greatly — and the amount of blood doesn't necessarily correspond to how much of the placenta has separated from the inner wall of the uterus.

Other signs and symptoms of placental abruption may include:

- Abdominal pain
- Back pain
- Uterine tenderness
- Rapid uterine contractions

If you experience any of these signs or symptoms, contact your health care provider right away or seek emergency care.

Causes: The exact cause of placental abruption is often unknown.

Rarely, trauma or injury to the abdomen — from an auto accident or fall, for example — causes placental abruption. In other rare cases, placental abruption is caused by an unusually short umbilical cord or rapid loss of amniotic fluid, the fluid that surrounds and protects the baby in the uterus.

Risk factors: High blood pressure (hypertension) in pregnancy is the most common condition associated with placental abruption. That's true whether the high blood pressure first developed during pregnancy or was present before conception. Maternal blood-clotting disorders also increase the risk of placental abruption.

Placental abruption appears to be more common in women older than 40 and those who have:

- Diabetes
- A multiple pregnancy
- An unusually large amount of amniotic fluid
- Numerous previous deliveries

Lifestyle factors play a role as well. Placental abruption is more common in women who smoke and those who abuse alcohol and drugs such as cocaine during pregnancy.

If you experience placental abruption, there's at least a 10 percent chance that the condition will recur in a subsequent pregnancy. After two episodes of placental abruption, the chance of recurrence increases to more than 20 percent.

When to seek medical advice?: If you have placental abruption, prompt treatment is essential. Contact your health care provider right away or seek emergency care if you experience signs or symptoms of placental abruption, including:

- Vaginal bleeding
- New back pain
- Abdominal pain
- Rapid uterine contractions, often coming one right after another

Screening and diagnosis: If your health care provider suspects placental abruption, he or she will check for uterine tenderness or rigidity. Your health care provider may do blood tests or an ultrasound to help identify possible sources of bleeding. Diagnosis is based on the overall clinical circumstances. Often, placental abruption can't be confirmed until after delivery — when the placenta is delivered with an attached blood clot.

Complications: Placental abruption can cause life-threatening problems for you and your baby. Without prompt treatment, maternal blood loss may lead to shock. Your baby may be deprived of oxygen and nutrients. Sometimes, decreased oxygen to the brain leads to later neurological or behavioral problems. In severe cases, the baby may not survive. Blood loss may be a concern after delivery, too. If bleeding from the site of the placental attachment can't be controlled after the baby is born, emergency removal of the uterus (hysterectomy) may be needed

Treatment: If your health care provider suspects placental abruption, treatment depends on your condition, the baby's condition and the stage of the pregnancy.

If the abruption seems mild, if your baby's heart rate is normal, and if it's too soon for the baby to be born, you may be hospitalised for close monitoring. If the bleeding stops and your baby's condition is stable, your health care provider may prescribe bed rest at home. In some circumstances, you may be given medication to help your baby's lungs mature — in case early delivery becomes necessary.

If you're 36 weeks or more into your pregnancy and placental abruption is minimal, a closely monitored vaginal delivery may be possible. If the abruption progresses or jeopardises your health or your baby's health, you'll need an immediate delivery — usually by Caesarean section. If you experience severe bleeding, you may need a blood transfusion.

Prevention: You can't prevent placental abruption — but you can decrease certain risk factors. Don't drink alcohol, smoke or take illicit drugs during pregnancy. If you have high blood pressure or diabetes, work with your health care provider to control your condition.

If you've had a placental abruption, talk to your health care provider before conceiving again. When you become pregnant, your health care provider will carefully monitor your condition to make sure your pregnancy is progressing normally

Preeclampsia

Preeclampsia is a common problem during pregnancy, affecting up to one in seven pregnant women around the world. This condition is defined by high blood pressure and excess protein in the urine after 20 weeks of pregnancy. It may also be called toxemia or pregnancy-induced hypertension.

In the United States, preeclampsia (pree-i-KLAMP-see-uh) is usually mild. But, left untreated, it can lead to serious, even deadly complications for you and your unborn baby. Globally, preeclampsia and other high blood pressure disorders during pregnancy are a leading cause of maternal and infant illness and death.

The only cure for preeclampsia is delivery of your baby. After your baby is born, blood pressure usually returns to normal within a few days. So delivery is the obvious solution when preeclampsia is found near the end of your pregnancy, which is typically the case. However, if you're diagnosed earlier, treatment is trickier.

You and your doctor will be faced with the delicate task of prolonging your pregnancy to allow your baby more time to mature, without putting you or your baby at risk of serious complications.

Signs and symptoms: The signs of preeclampsia are elevated blood pressure (hypertension) and the presence of excess protein in your urine (proteinuria) after 20 weeks of pregnancy. Your health care provider may identify these signs of preeclampsia at one of your regular prenatal visits.

Other signs and symptoms aren't always noticeable, but you may experience:

- Severe headaches
- Changes in vision, including temporary loss of vision, blurred vision or light sensitivity
- Upper abdominal pain, usually under the ribs on the right side
- Unexplained anxiety
- Nausea or vomiting
- Dizziness
- Decreased urine output

Swelling (edema), particularly in the face and hands, was once considered a primary sign of preeclampsia. But because swelling also occurs in a large number of normal pregnancies, it's no longer considered a reliable indicator. However, sudden weight gain — typically more than two pounds a week or six pounds a month — may be an early sign of preeclampsia.

Preeclampsia can develop gradually or come on suddenly. It may occur during the last half of pregnancy, during delivery or even in the first few days after your baby is born. But it's most common in the last few weeks of pregnancy and usually resolves soon after delivery. In some cases, it takes a few days or weeks for blood pressure to completely return to normal.

Other high blood pressure disorders during pregnancy: Doctors classify preeclampsia as one of four high blood pressure disorders that can occur during pregnancy. The other three are:

- *Gestational hypertension:* Women with gestational hypertension have high blood pressure, but no excess protein in their urine. In most cases, the high blood pressure is mild and occurs in the later stages of pregnancy. If you are diagnosed with gestational hypertension, your doctor will continue checking for proteinuria, which signals that gestational hypertension has progressed into preeclampsia. About one in four women with gestational hypertension go on to develop preeclampsia.

- *Chronic hypertension:* Chronic hypertension is high blood pressure that appears before 20 weeks of pregnancy or lasts more than 12 weeks after delivery. In some cases, women know they have chronic high blood pressure before they become pregnant. But, in many cases, women with long-standing high blood pressure are not evaluated for the problem before they become pregnant. Their high blood pressure is discovered only during prenatal care, but because blood pressure is often low in early pregnancy, it may not be detected initially. Chronic high blood pressure isn't caused by pregnancy. If it doesn't disappear after delivery, you probably had it all along and were never diagnosed.

- *Preeclampsia superimposed on chronic hypertension:* This is a fancy term for women who have chronic high blood pressure before they become pregnant and then go on to develop protein in their urine. This term is also used for women who have high blood pressure and protein in the urine before pregnancy, if there is a marked increase in either problem during the last half of pregnancy.

If you are diagnosed with any of these three high blood pressure disorders, your doctor will closely monitor you and your baby. He or she will also explain possible risks and treatment options. These disorders have some similarities with preeclampsia, but they're not exactly the same.

Causes: Preeclampsia used to be called toxemia because it

was thought to be caused by a toxin in a pregnant woman's bloodstream. Today, doctors and researchers know preeclampsia isn't caused by a toxin.

They've replaced this debunked theory with lots of other theories about what may cause preeclampsia, but there's no clear answer yet, despite extensive research. Possible causes include:

- Insufficient blood flow to your uterus
- Injury to your blood vessels
- Damage to the lining of your blood vessels
- A disruption in the hormones that maintain your blood vessels
- A mistake by your immune system
- Poor diet
- Lack of magnesium or calcium

Risk factors: The biggest risk factor for preeclampsia is simply being pregnant. Additional risk factors include:

- *History of preeclampsia:* A personal history of preeclampsia or family history of preeclampsia increases your risk of developing the condition.
- *First pregnancy:* Your chances of developing preeclampsia are greater if this is your first pregnancy, your first pregnancy with a new partner, or your first pregnancy in 10 years or more.
- *Age:* Your risk of preeclampsia increases if you're younger than 20 or older than 35 at the time of pregnancy.
- *Obesity:* Having a pre-pregnancy body mass index (BMI) greater than 30 is a risk factor for preeclampsia.
- *Multiple pregnancy:* Preeclampsia is more common in women who are carrying twins, triplets or more.
- *History of certain conditions:* Having certain conditions before you become pregnant can be a risk factor for preeclampsia. This includes chronic high blood pressure, diabetes, kidney disease or connective tissue disease — such as rheumatoid arthritis or lupus.

In a 2006 study, pregnant women who had high levels of

two specific proteins in their blood were found to be more likely to develop preeclampsia than were other women. These proteins interfere with the growth and function of blood vessels. Research to confirm the findings is needed — but the discovery suggests that a blood test may one day serve as an effective screening tool for preeclampsia.

When to seek medical advice?: When you're pregnant, you're likely to experience some discomfort. Headaches, nausea, and aches and pains can be common. It's difficult to know when new symptoms are just part of being pregnant and when they may indicate a serious problem — especially if it's your first pregnancy. The best policy is to trust your instincts and see your health care provider if you just don't feel right.

Call your health care provider right away if you have severe headaches, blurred vision or severe pain in your abdomen. But don't take a wait-and-see approach to other ailments. Serious complications of preeclampsia can occur even before symptoms of preeclampsia, and you don't get any points for toughing it out until the situation is serious.

Screening and diagnosis: Preeclampsia usually shows up unexpectedly during a routine prenatal blood pressure check and urine test. So, it's important to seek regular prenatal care throughout your pregnancy.

You'll be diagnosed with preeclampsia if you have an elevated blood pressure and protein in your urine after 20 weeks of pregnancy. Normal blood pressure readings for pregnant women are below 130/85 millimeters of mercury (mm Hg). A blood pressure reading of 140/90 mm Hg or higher is considered above the normal range. However, a single high blood pressure reading doesn't mean you have preeclampsia. If you have one reading in the abnormal range — or a reading that is substantially higher than your normal blood pressure — your health care provider will closely observe your numbers. You may also be asked to come in for additional blood pressure readings and urinary protein measurements.

If you do have preeclampsia, you health care provider may

want to do some blood tests to see how well your liver and kidneys are functioning and to see if your blood has the normal number of cells that help blood clot (platelets). Your health care provider may also recommend close monitoring of your baby's growth — usually using ultrasound. This test combines high-frequency sound waves and computer processing to generate pictures of the inside of your uterus.

You may need a nonstress test (NST) or biophysical profile to make sure your baby is getting enough oxygen and nourishment, especially as you approach your due date. A nonstress test is just that — a noninvasive test that causes no stress to your baby. In fact, it shouldn't be stressful for you either. The test usually takes less than 30 minutes and requires no hospitalization. It's a simple procedure that checks how often your baby moves and how much his or her heart rate increases with movement. A biophysical profile combines an ultrasound with a nonstress test to provide more information about your baby's breathing, tone, movement and the volume of amniotic fluid in your uterus.

Complications: Most women with preeclampsia go on to deliver healthy babies. But preeclampsia is a serious condition that can lead to two serious conditions and some problems for your baby. The more severe your preeclampsia and the earlier it occurs in your pregnancy, the greater the risks for you and your baby.

HELLP syndrome: HELLP syndrome is one of two serious complications of preeclampsia. HELLP stands for:

- Hemolysis — the destruction of red blood cells
- Elevated Liver Enzymes
- Low Platelet Count

Symptoms of HELLP include nausea and vomiting, headache and upper right abdominal pain. This syndrome occurs in up to 12 percent of women with preeclampsia, and it can rapidly become life-threatening. It can cause liver failure and problems with blood clotting (coagulation), which may pose a high risk of death to you or your baby. This syndrome is particularly dangerous because it can occur before you exhibit signs or symptoms of preeclampsia.

Eclampsia: The second serious complication that can develop is eclampsia — which is basically preeclampsia plus seizures. This life-threatening condition can develop when signs and symptoms of preeclampsia aren't controlled. Eclampsia can permanently damage your vital organs, including your brain, liver and kidneys. If left untreated, the condition can cause coma, brain damage and death to you or your baby.

Preeclampsia got its name because it was first identified as the condition that led to eclampsia. But now doctors realise that this progression isn't inevitable. In fact, eclampsia is rare in most countries.

The warning signs and symptoms of eclampsia include:
- Pain in the upper right side of your abdomen
- Severe headache
- Vision problems, including seeing flashing lights
- Change in mental status, such as decreased alertness

Problems for your baby: Preeclampsia affects the arteries carrying blood to your placenta. If your placenta doesn't get enough blood, your baby may receive less oxygen and nutrients. This can cause slow growth or a low birth weight. Preeclampsia is also a leading cause of preterm birth.

In addition, preeclampsia increases the risk of placental abruption— in which the placenta separates from the inner wall of the uterus before delivery. Severe abruption can cause heavy bleeding, which can cause the mother to go into shock. This condition is rare, but it's life-threatening for mother and baby. It requires immediate medical attention.

Rarely, preeclampsia may affect the fetus earlier and more severely than it affects the mother. So it's important for your doctor to monitor your unborn baby carefully even if your preeclampsia seems mild.

Treatment: The only cure for preeclampsia is delivery. After delivery, blood pressure usually returns to normal within a few days. So, delivery is always beneficial for the mother, who is at increased risk of seizures, placental abruption and severe bleeding (hemorrhage) until her blood pressure goes down.

Of course, delivery may not be the best thing for your baby, if it's too early in your pregnancy. So your doctor will consider how far along your baby is in terms of development before inducing labour. Ideally, your doctor will try to manage your condition so that you can deliver your baby after you've reached 36 weeks of pregnancy. In more severe cases, it may not be possible to wait, and you may need to undergo induction or Caesarean birth earlier.

Bed rest: Buying time for baby to grow: If you aren't near the very end of your pregnancy and you have a mild case of preeclampsia, your doctor may try to delay delivery to give your baby more time to grow and mature. In this situation, your condition may be managed at home with bed rest and regular monitoring of your blood pressure.

The rules for bed rest depend on your individual situation. You may need to lie in bed, only sitting and standing when necessary. Or you may be advised to sit on the couch or in bed and to limit your activities. Bed rest can increase blood flow to your placenta and lower blood pressure in general, so it can be an effective way to give your baby extra time to mature. Your health care provider may want to see you a few times a week, to check your blood pressure, urine protein levels and the status of your baby.

A more severe case of preeclampsia often requires bed rest in a hospital. In the hospital, you'll undergo regular nonstress tests or biophysical profiles to monitor your baby's well-being. You may also have ultrasound exams to measure the volume of amniotic fluid. If the amount is too low, it's a sign that the blood supply to the baby has been inadequate, and you may need to deliver your baby.

Medications: Helpful for you and your baby: Your doctor may recommend medications to treat high blood pressure if you experience a dangerous increase in blood pressure. These medications can be lifesaving. However, lowering your blood pressure doesn't really treat the source of the problem. Delivery is still necessary to cure preeclampsia.

Corticosteroids may also be beneficial for women with preeclampsia or HELLP syndrome. Potent corticosteroid medications can temporarily improve liver and platelet functioning in women with severe preeclampsia. As a result, these medications may help prolong pregnancy in situations where the baby is too young for delivery in terms of gestational development.

Corticosteroids may serve another purpose, too. They can help make your baby's lungs more mature in as little as 48 hours. Underdeveloped lungs are one of the biggest problems facing premature infants. So corticosteroids can be an important step in helping an immature baby prepare for life outside of the uterus.

Delivery: The ultimate cure for preeclampsia: Many cases of preeclampsia are discovered at the very end of pregnancy, so they can be treated by inducing labour right away. If you have preeclampsia, your doctor probably won't let you go beyond 40 weeks of pregnancy because of the increased risks to your baby. The readiness of your cervix — whether it's beginning to open (dilate), thin (efface) and soften (ripen)— also may be a factor in determining whether or when labour will be induced.

In more severe cases, it may not be possible to consider your baby's gestational age or the readiness of your cervix. Your doctor will recommend inducing labour or performing a Caesarean birth if your health or the health of your baby is at risk or if your blood pressure continues to rise. In these cases, the benefits of delivering the baby early outweigh the risks of waiting. During delivery, you may be given magnesium sulfate intravenously to increase uterine blood flow and prevent seizures.

Prevention: There's currently no known way to prevent preeclampsia. Eating less salt or changing your activities during pregnancy doesn't reduce the risk. The best way to take care of yourself — and your baby— is to seek early and regular prenatal care. If preeclampsia is detected early, you and your doctor can work together to prevent complications and make the best choices for you and your baby.

Researchers are studying the possible preventive effects of

exercise, good nutrition, low-dose aspirin, calcium supplements and antioxidants. In a preliminary 2006 study, women who took multivitamins and maintained a healthy weight before conception reduced the risk of developing preeclampsia during pregnancy by more than 70 percent compared with women of a healthy weight who didn't take multivitamins or with women who took multivitamins but were overweight before conception.

Several earlier studies suggested that specific nutritional supplements could prevent preeclampsia, but these studies haven't stood the test of time. Although a healthy weight before pregnancy has clear benefits for both mother and baby, more research is needed to determine the preventive effects of multivitamins and other nutritional supplements.

Coping skills: Discovering that you have a condition that can affect the health of your unborn child can be downright terrifying. If you are diagnosed with preeclampsia late in your pregnancy, you may be surprised and scared by the news that you will be induced right away.

If you are diagnosed earlier in your pregnancy, you may have many hours of bed rest — way too much time — to worry about the health of your baby-to-be.

You'll probably feel better if you learn as much as you can about your condition. In addition to talking to your doctor, do some research. Or ask your doctor to put you in touch with other women who have had preeclampsia.

On the other hand, if reading about preeclampsia and its possible complications is just making you more nervous and worried, find a distraction. Make sure you understand when to call your doctor, and then seek out something else to occupy your time.

Coping with bed rest: For the first few hours, bed rest may seem wonderful. You have permission to rest, and your family is waiting on you hand and foot. But the reality of life in bed, waiting and worrying, is often not so wonderful.

In fact, if you don't feel sick, you may feel frustrated by this forced vacation, especially if you haven't had time to finish preparations for your baby's arrival.

Make the best of the situation by focusing on the fact that you're doing what's best for you and your baby. After all, your baby's well-being is far more important than stenciling the nursery or picking out the perfect going-home-from-the-hospital outfit.

To make bed rest tolerable, try these tips:

- *Make sure you understand the ground rules:* Ask your health care provider exactly what your restrictions are. What position should you use while lying down? Can you sit up at times? If so, for how long? Is there any other type of physical activity allowed?

- *Prepare your resting room:* Whether you choose to spend your time in your bedroom or in the living room, set up your surroundings so everything you need is within reach from the bed or couch. If you need help arranging your area, ask your partner or a family member.

- *Organise your day:* The hours will pass more quickly if you have some sort of routine. Schedule specific times to phone the office, watch television and read. It may help to stick to some parts of your normal schedule, such as lunchtime and lights out.

- *Plan for your baby's arrival:* Read about newborn care — how to bathe, dress, breast-feed and soothe your baby. Consider purchasing newborn necessities, either online or from catalogs. If you have access to a computer, you can also use the Internet to find tips and advice from other moms on bed rest.

- *Keep busy:* Use your time to balance the checkbook, organise old photo albums, catch up on thank-you notes or fill out health insurance paperwork for your baby in advance. Take up a new hobby, such as making a scrapbook, painting or knitting. Or learn relaxation and visualization techniques. They'll help not only during bed rest but also during labour and delivery.

8

Diagnosis of Pregnancy

SYMPTOMS AND SIGNS; BIOLOGICAL TESTS

Outward early indications of pregnancy are missed menstrual periods, morning nausea, and fullness and tenderness of the breasts; but the positive and certain signs of gestation are the sounds of the fetal heartbeat, which are audible with a stethoscope between the 16th and the 20th week of pregnancy; ultrasound images of the growing fetus, which can be observed throughout pregnancy; and fetal movements, which usually occur by the 18th to the 20th week of pregnancy.

Persons who note their body temperature upon awakening, as many women do who wish to know when they are ovulating, may observe continued elevation of the temperature curve well beyond the time of the missed period; this is strongly suggestive of pregnancy. During the early months of pregnancy, women may notice that they urinate frequently, because of pressure of the enlarging uterus on the bladder; feel tired and drowsy; dislike foods that were previously palatable; have a sense of pelvic heaviness; and are subject to vomiting (which can be severe) and to pulling pains in the sides of the abdomen, as the growing uterus stretches the round ligaments that help support it, singly or together. Most of these symptoms subside as pregnancy progresses. The signs and symptoms of pregnancy are so definite by the 12th week that the diagnosis is seldom a problem.

Biological tests for pregnancy depend upon the production by the placenta (the temporary organ that develops in the womb for the nourishing of the embryo and the elimination of its wastes) of chorionic gonadotropin, an ovary-stimulating hormone. In practice, the tests have an accuracy of about 95 percent, although false-negative tests may run as high as 20 percent in a series of cases. False-negative reports are frequently obtained during late pregnancy when the secretion of chorionic gonadotropin normally decreases.

The possibility not only of false-negative but also of false-positive tests makes the tests, at best, probable rather than absolute evidence of the presence or absence of pregnancy. Chorionic gonadotropin in a woman's blood or urine indicates only that she is harbouring living placental tissue. It does not tell anything about the condition of the fetus. In fact, the greatest production of chorionic gonadotropin occurs in certain placental abnormalities and disorders that can develop in the absence of a fetus.

Tests using immature mice (the Aschheim-Zondek test) and immature rats have been found to be extremely accurate. Tests using rabbits (the Friedman test) have been largely replaced by the more rapid and less expensive frog and toad tests.

The use of the female South African claw-toed tree toad, *Xenopus laevis*, is based on the discovery that this animal will ovulate and extrude visible eggs within a few hours after it has received an injection of a few millilitres of urine from a pregnant woman. The male common frog, *Rana pipiens*, will extrude spermatozoa when treated in the same way. Both of these tests are considered somewhat unsatisfactory because false-positive reactions are not uncommon.

Several immunological reaction tests in common use are based upon the inhibition of hemagglutination (clotting of red cells). A positive test is obtained when human chorionic gonadotropin (HCG) in the woman's urine or blood is added to human chorionic gonadotropin antiserum (rabbit blood serum containing antibodies to HCG) in the presence of particles (or red blood cells) coated with human chorionic gonadotropin. The hormone from the woman will inhibit the combination of coated particles and antibody, and agglutination does not occur. If there is no chorionic gonadotropin in her urine, agglutination will occur and the test is negative.

Several "signs" noted by the physician during an examination will suggest that a patient may be in the early months of pregnancy. Darkening of the areola of the breast (the small, coloured ring around the nipple) and prominence of the sebaceous glands around the nipple (Montgomery's glands); purplish-red discoloration of the vulvar, vaginal, and cervical tissues; softening of the cervix and of the lower part of the uterus and, of course, enlargement and softening of the uterus itself are suggestive but not necessarily proof of pregnancy.

CONDITIONS THAT MAY BE MISTAKEN FOR PREGNANCY

Other conditions may confuse the diagnosis of pregnancy. Absence of menstruation can be caused by chronic illness, by emotional or endocrine disturbances, by fear of pregnancy, or by a desire to be pregnant. Nausea and vomiting may be of gastrointestinal or psychic origin. Tenderness of the breasts can be due to a hormonal disturbance.

Any condition that causes pelvic congestion, such as a pelvic tumour, may cause duskiness of the genital tissues. At times a soft tumour of the uterus may simulate a pregnancy. The question of pregnancy may be raised if the woman does not menstruate regularly; the absence of other symptoms and signs of gestation indicates that she is not pregnant. There are rare ovarian and uterine tumours that produce false-positive pregnancy tests. It may be difficult for the physician to exclude pregnancy on the basis of an examination if the uterus is tipped back and difficult to feel, or if it is enlarged by a tumour within it. If other signs of pregnancy are absent, however, and the tests for pregnancy are negative, pregnancy can most likely be ruled out.

Childless women who greatly desire a baby sometimes suffer from false or spurious pregnancy (pseudocyesis). They stop menstruating, have morning nausea, "feel life," and have abdominal enlargement caused by fat and intestinal gas. At "term" they may have "labour pains." Signs of pregnancy are absent. Treatment is by psychotherapy. Menopausal women often fear pregnancy when their periods stop; information that they show no signs of pregnancy usually reassures them. Retained uterine secretions of bloody or watery fluid, caught above a blocked mouth of the uterus (cervix), prevent menstruation, cause softening and enlargement of the uterus, and may cause the patient to wonder whether she is pregnant. There are no other signs of pregnancy, and the hard cervix, closed by scar tissue, explains the problem.

THE UTERUS AND THE DEVELOPMENT OF THE PLACENTA

The uterus is a thick-walled, pear-shaped organ measuring seven centimetres (about 2.75 inches) in length and weighing 30 grams (about one ounce) in an unpregnant woman in her later teens. It has a buttonlike lower end, the cervix, that merges with the bulbous larger portion, called the corpus.

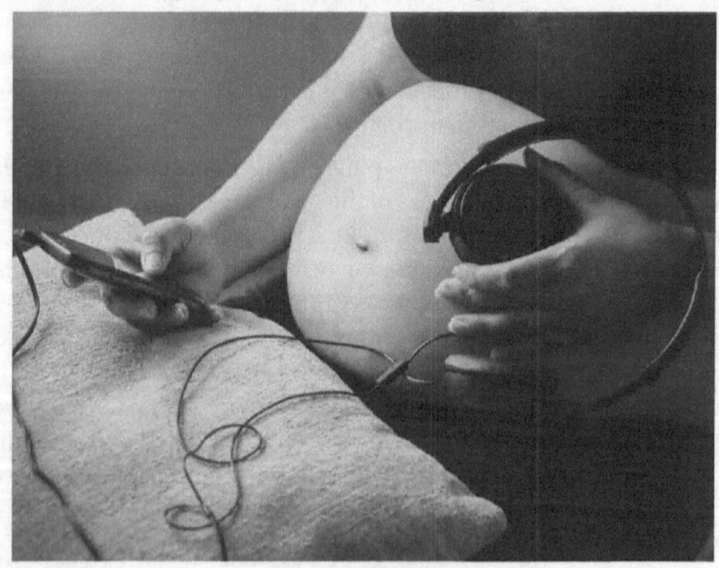

True or False: Pregnancy Myths

The corpus comprises approximately three-fourths of the uterus. There is a flat, triangular-shaped cavity within the uterus. At term, the uterus is a large, thin-walled, hollow, elastic, fluid-filled cylinder measuring approximately 30 centimetres (about

12 inches) in length, weighing approximately 1,200 grams (2.6 pounds), and having a capacity of 4,000 to 5,000 millilitres (4.2 to 5.3 quarts).

The greater size of the uterus as a result of pregnancy is due to a marked increase in the number of muscle fibres, blood vessels, nerves, and lymphatic vessels in the uterine wall. There is also a five- to tenfold increase in the size of the individual muscle fibre and marked enlargement in the diameters of the blood and lymph vessels.

During the first few weeks of pregnancy, the shape of the uterus is unchanged, but the organ becomes gradually softer. By the 14th week it forms a flattened or oblate spheroid. The fibrous cervix becomes remarkably softer and acquires a protective mucus plug within its cavity, but otherwise it changes little before labour. The lower part of the corpus, the isthmus, first becomes elongated and then, as the uterine contents demand more space, stretches and unfolds to form a bowl-shaped formation called the lower uterine segment. The fibrous nature of the cervix causes it to resist this unfolding action.

The uterine wall is stretched and thinned during pregnancy by the growing conceptus, as the whole product of conception is called, and by the fluid that surrounds it. By term, this process converts the uterus into an elastic, fluid-filled cylinder. It is only late in pregnancy that the cervix gradually thins out and softens; during labour it dilates for passage of the infant.

As pregnancy progresses, the uterus rises out of the pelvis and fills the abdominal cavity. It is top-heavy near term so that it falls forward and, because of the large bowel on the left side, rotates to the right. It presses on the diaphragm and pushes the other organs aside. The uterus may sink downward in the pelvis several weeks before term in a process that is known as lightening or dropping. This occurs as the fetal head descends into the pelvis. In some women, particularly those who have borne children, lightening does not occur until the onset of labour. Lightening may be impossible in women who have an abnormally small pelvis, an oversized fetus, or a fetus lying in an abnormal position.

For a short time after fertilization, the conceptus, a minute bubblelike structure called a blastocyst, lies unattached in the uterine cavity. The cells that will become the embryo (the embryonic disk) form a thickened layer on one side of the bubble. Elsewhere, the walls of the bubble consist of a single layer of cells; these cells are the trophoblast, which has a special ability to attach to and invade the uterine wall. The trophoblast plays an important role later in the development of the placenta or afterbirth. The conceptus makes contact with the uterine lining about the fifth or sixth day after conception. After contact the blastocyst collapses to form a rounded disk with the embryonic mass on the surface and the trophoblast against the endometrium (uterine lining). The part of the trophoblast that is in contact with the endometrium grows into and invades the maternal tissue. Concomitant disintegration of the endometrium allows the conceptus to sink into the uterine lining.

Soon the entire blastocyst is buried in the endometrium. Proliferation of the trophoblast over the part of the collapsed bubble that is opposite the embryo is part of the implantation procedure that helps to cover the blastocyst. After a few days, a cavity forms that bears the same relation to the embryonic disk that the blastocyst cavity did before; this cavity will become the fluid-filled chorionic cavity containing the embryo. Ultimately it will contain the amniotic fluid that surrounds the fetus, the fetus itself, and the umbilical cord.

The body stalk, which will become the umbilical cord, then begins to separate the embryo from the syncytiotrophoblast, the outer layer of the trophoblast lying against the endometrium; the inner lining of the trophoblast is called cytotrophoblast. As the syncytiotrophoblast advances into the endometrium, it surrounds minute branches of the uterine arteries that contain maternal blood. Erosion of the endometrium about these blood sinuses allows them to open into the small cavities in the trophoblast. The cytotrophoblast, which lines the cavity, forms fingers of proliferating cells extending into the syncytiotrophoblast. After the placenta is developed, these fingers will be the cores of the rootlike placental villi, structures that will draw nutrients and oxygen from the maternal blood that bathes them. This is the first step in uteroplacental circulation, which supplies the fetus with all of the sustenance necessary for life and growth and removes waste products from it. During the third week of pregnancy, the syncytiotrophoblast forms a single layer of cells covering the growing villi and lining the syncytial lacunae or small cavities between the villi. The conceptus is buried in the endometrium, and its whole surface is covered at this time by developing villi. The greater part of the chorionic wall is now cytotrophoblast. Fingers of cytotrophoblast in the form of cell masses extend into the syncytial layer. Soon thereafter, a layer of connective tissue, or mesoderm, grows into the villi, which now form branches as they spread out into the blood-filled spaces in the endometrium adjacent to the conceptus.

By the end of the third week, the chorionic villi that form the outer surface of the chorionic sac are covered by a thick layer of cytotrophoblast and have a connective tissue core within which embryonic blood vessels are beginning to develop. The vessels, which arise from the yolk sac, connect with the primitive vascular system in the embryo. As growth progresses the layer of cytotrophoblast begins to regress. It disappears by the fifth month of pregnancy.

The layer of endometrium closest to the encroaching conceptus forms, with remnants of the invading syncytiotrophoblast, a thin plate of cells known as the decidua basalis, the maternal component of the mature placenta; it is cast off when the placenta is expelled. The fetal part of the placenta—the villi and their contained blood vessels—is separated from the decidua basalis by a lakelike body of fluid blood. This pool was created by coalescence of the intervillous spaces. The intervillous spaces in turn were formed from the syncytial lacunae in the young conceptus. Maternal blood enters this blood mass from the branches of the uterine arteries. The pool is drained by the uterine veins. It is so choked by intermingling villi and their branches that its continuity is lost on gross inspection.

The chorionic cavity contains the fluid in which the embryo floats. As its shell or outer surface becomes larger, the decidua capsularis, which is that part of the endometrium that has grown over the side of the conceptus away from the embryo (i.e., the abembryonic side) after implantation, becomes thinner. After 12 weeks or so, the villi on this side, which is the side directed toward the uterine cavity, disappear, leaving the smooth chorion, now called the chorion laeve. The chorion frondosum is that part of the conceptus that forms as the villi grow larger on the side of the chorionic shell next to the uterine wall. The discus-shaped placenta develops from the chorion frondosum and the decidua basalis.

At term, the normal placenta is a disk-shaped structure approximately 16 to 20 centimetres (about six to seven inches) in diameter, three or four centimetres (about 1.2–1.6 inches) in thickness at its thickest part, and weighing between 500 and 1,000 grams (1.1 and 2.2 pounds). It is thinner at its margins, where it is joined to the membrane-like chorion which spreads out over the whole inner surface of the uterus and contains the fetus and the amniotic fluid.

The amnion, a thinner membrane, is adherent to and covers the inner surface of the chorion. The inner or fetal surface of the placenta is shiny, smooth, and traversed by a number of branching fetal blood vessels that come together at the point—usually the centre of the placenta—where the umbilical cord attaches. The maternal or uterine side of the placenta, covered by the thin, flaky decidua basalis, a cast-off part of the uterine lining, is rough and purplish-red, and has a raw appearance.

When the placenta is cut across, its interior is seen to be made of a soft, crepelike or spongy matrix from which semisolid or clotted blood, caught when it is separated from the uterine wall to which it was attached, can be squeezed. Detailed examination shows that the villi and their branches form an arborescent (treelike) mass within the huge blood lake of the intervillous space. Anchoring villi extend outward from the fetal side and fuse with the decidua basalis to hold the organ's shape. Others, algaelike, float freely in the blood lake. Dividing partitions, formed from the trophoblast shell, project into the intervillous space from the decidual side. They divide the placenta into 15 or 20 compartments, which are called cotyledons.

Maternal blood flows from the uterine vessels into the trophoblast-lined intervillous blood lake. Within each villus is a blood vessel network that is part of the fetal circulatory system. Blood within the villous vessel is circulated by the fetal heart. The blood vessel wall, the connective tissue of the villous core, and the syncytiotrophoblast covering the villus lie between the fetal and the maternal bloodstreams. This is known as the placental barrier. As pregnancy progresses, the fetal blood vessels become larger, the connective tissue stretches over them, and the syncytiotrophoblastic layer becomes fragmentary. As a result, the placental barrier becomes much thinner. Normally, blood cells and bacteria do not pass through it, but nutrients, water, salt, viruses, hormones, and many other substances, including many drugs, can filter across it.

UTERINE TUBES

One of the two uterine tubes is the pathway down which the ripe ovum travels on its way to the uterus or womb. The spermatozoa from the male migrate up the tube, and it is there that they meet the ovum and fertilization occurs. During the first few days after fertilization the zygote, or fertilized egg, moves downward in the tube toward the uterus. While it is lying free in the tubal canal, the young conceptus is nourished by secretions from the tube. After the fertilized egg (or conceptus) passes into the uterus, the tube ceases to play any part in the pregnancy; in fact, the only function the tube has is carried out during those few days before, during, and after conception. As pregnancy goes on, the tube gradually enlarges, however, and contains more blood, as do all the pelvic organs; some of its cells may show a reaction, called a decidual reaction, to the hormones of pregnancy. As the uterus increases in size, the tubes stretch upward with it until they become two greatly enlarged elongated strands, one on each side of the uterus.

Vagina

The pinkish tan colour of the lining of the vagina gradually takes on a bluish cast during the early months of pregnancy as a result of the dilation of the blood vessels in the vaginal wall; later the vaginal wall tends to become a purplish red colour as the blood vessels become further engorged. The cells of the vaginal mucosa increase in size. Added numbers of these cells peel off the surface of the mucosa and mix with the increased vaginal fluid. This produces a profuse vaginal secretion. Thickening, softening, and relaxation of the loosely folded, succulent lining of the vagina and the sodden tissues beneath it greatly increase distensibility and capacity of the vaginal cavity; this is a process that partially prepares the birth canal for the passage through it of the large fetal mass.

External genital structures

Changes in the external genitalia are similar to those in the vagina. The tissues become first softened and more succulent and later extremely fragile, as an increasing amount of blood and fluid collects in them. They take on a purplish red colour because of increased blood supply. Darkening of the vulvar skin, frequently seen during pregnancy, is particularly common among women of Mediterranean ethnic groups.

Other pelvic tissues

The pelvic blood vessels and lymph channels become larger and longer. They develop new branches adequate to transport the greatly increased amounts of blood and tissue fluid that accumulate in the uterus and the other pelvic organs during pregnancy. Congestion and engorgement of blood in the pelvis, both within and without the uterus, are characteristic of pregnancy.

Changes in the muscles, ligaments, and other supporting tissues of the pelvis begin early in pregnancy and become progressively more pronounced as pregnancy continues. These changes are induced by the greatly increased hormonal levels in the mother's blood that characterize pregnancy. Before labour starts, the pelvic supporting tissues must have sufficient elasticity and strength to permit the uterus to grow out of the pelvis and yet support it. The muscles must be soft and elastic enough during delivery so that they can stretch apart and not obstruct the baby's birth.

Softening and greater elasticity is brought about not only by the growth of new tissue but also by congestion and retained fluid within the tissues themselves.

The bones forming the mother's pelvis show relatively few changes during pregnancy. Loosening of the joint between the pubic bones in front and of the joints between the sacrum and the pelvis in back occurs as a response to the hormone called relaxin, which is produced by the ovary. Although relaxin, which causes marked separation of the pelvic joints in some animals, usually has too slight an effect in human beings to be noticed, softening of the attachments between the bones may be sufficient to cause a few women considerable distress. The strain on the joint between the sacrum and the spine becomes greater near term when the woman tilts her pelvis forward and bends the upper part of her body backward to compensate for the weight of the heavy uterus. When relaxation is excessive, the woman suffers from backache and difficulty in walking. If it is extreme, she may have a waddling gait. Relaxation of the pelvic joints does not disappear quickly after delivery; it accounts for much of the backache that women with new babies experience.

The mother's bones show no structural change if her calcium reserve and intake are normal. If her reserve and intake are not adequate, the fetus may draw so much calcium from her bones that the bones become soft and deformed. This condition is rarely seen, except in areas of the world where extreme poverty and serious calcium deficiency are major problems.

Breasts

The earliest changes in the breasts during pregnancy are an exaggeration of the frequently experienced premenstrual discomfort and fullness. The sensation is so specific for pregnancy that many women who have been pregnant before are made aware of their condition by the feeling that they have in their breasts. As pregnancy progresses the breasts become larger, the lightly pigmented area (areola) around each nipple becomes first florid or dusky in colour and then appreciably darker; during the later months the areola takes on a hue that is deep bronze or brownish black, depending on the woman's natural pigmentation. The veins beneath the skin over the breast become enlarged and more prominent. The small oily or sebaceous glands (glands of Montgomery) about the nipple become prominent.

These changes are due to the greatly increased levels of estrogen and progesterone in the woman's blood. These ovarian hormones also prepare the breast tissue for the action of the lactogenic (milk-causing) hormone, prolactin, produced by the pituitary gland. During the later part of pregnancy a milky fluid, colostrum, exudes from the ducts or can be expressed from them.

After delivery the decrease in estrogen and progesterone levels presumably permits the pituitary gland to release prolactin, which causes the breast to secrete milk. It is thought that the high hormonal levels inhibit the action or secretion of prolactin before delivery. Prolactin continues to be produced, and lactation usually continues, as long as the mother feeds her baby at the breast.

9

Anatomic and Physiologic Changes in Pregnancy

PHYSIOLOGY

Initiation

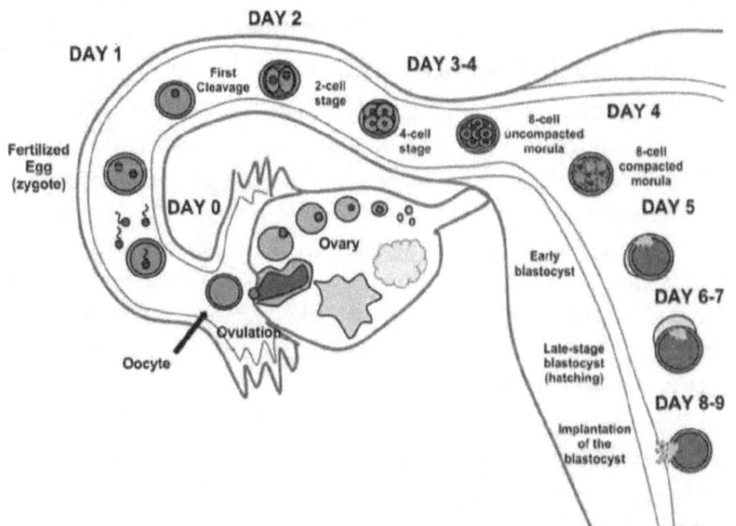

Fertilization and implantation in humans

Through an interplay of hormones that includes follicle stimulating hormone that stimulates folliculogenesis and oogenesis creates a mature egg cell, the female gamete. Fertilization is the event where the egg cell fuses with the male gamete, spermatozoon. After the point of fertilization, the fused product of the female and male gamete is referred to as a zygote or fertilized egg.

The fusion of female and male gametes usually occurs following the act of sexual intercourse. Pregnancy rates for sexual intercourse are highest during the menstrual cycle time from some 5 days before until 1 to 2 days after ovulation.

Fertilization can also occur by assisted reproductive technology such as artificial insemination and in vitro fertilisation. Fertilization (conception) is sometimes used as the initiation of pregnancy, with the derived age being termed fertilization age. Fertilization usually occurs about two weeks before the *next* expected menstrual period.

A third point in time is also considered by some people to be the true beginning of a pregnancy: This is time of implantation, when the future fetus attaches to the lining of the uterus. This is about a week to ten days after fertilization.

Development of embryo and fetus

The sperm and the egg cell, which has been released from one of the female's two ovaries, unite in one of the two Fallopian tubes. The fertilized egg, known as a zygote, then moves toward the uterus, a journey that can take up to a week to complete. Cell division begins approximately 24 to 36 hours after the female and male cells unite. Cell division continues at a rapid rate and the cells then develop into what is known as a blastocyst. The blastocyst arrives at the uterus and attaches to the uterine wall, a process known as implantation.

The development of the mass of cells that will become the infant is called embryogenesis during the first approximately ten weeks of gestation. During this time, cells begin to differentiate into the various body systems.

The basic outlines of the organ, body, and nervous systems are established. By the end of the embryonic stage, the beginnings of features such as fingers, eyes, mouth, and ears become visible.

Also during this time, there is development of structures important to the support of the embryo, including the placenta and umbilical cord. The placenta connects the developing embryo to the uterine wall to allow nutrient uptake, waste elimination, and gas exchange via the mother's blood supply. The umbilical cord is the connecting cord from the embryo or fetus to the placenta.

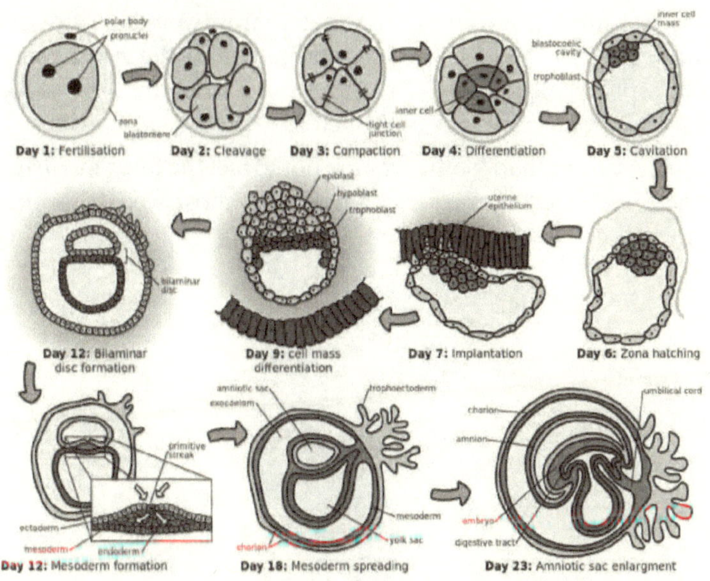

The initial stages of human embryogenesis

After about ten weeks of gestational age—which is the same as eight weeks after conception—the embryo becomes known as a fetus. At the beginning of the fetal stage, the risk of miscarriage decreases sharply. At this stage, a fetus is about 30 mm (1.2 inches) in length, the heartbeat is seen via ultrasound, and the fetus makes involuntary motions.

During continued fetal development, the early body systems, and structures that were established in the embryonic stage continue to develop. Sex organs begin to appear during the third month of gestation. The fetus continues to grow in both weight and length, although the majority of the physical growth occurs in the last weeks of pregnancy.

Electrical brain activity is first detected between the fifth and sixth week of gestation.

It is considered primitive neural activity rather than the beginning of conscious thought. Synapses begin forming at 17 weeks, and begin to multiply quickly at week 28 until 3 to 4 months after birth.

Although the fetus begins to move during the first trimester, it is not until the second trimester that movement, known as quickening, can be felt. This typically happens in the fourth month, more specifically in the 20th to 21st week, or by the 19th week if the woman has been pregnant before.

It is common for some women not to feel the fetus move until much later. During the second trimester, most women begin to wear maternity clothes.

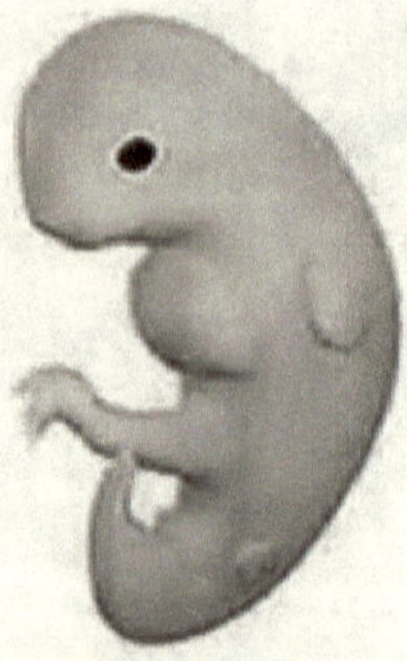

Embryo at 4 weeks after fertilization (gestational age of 6 weeks)

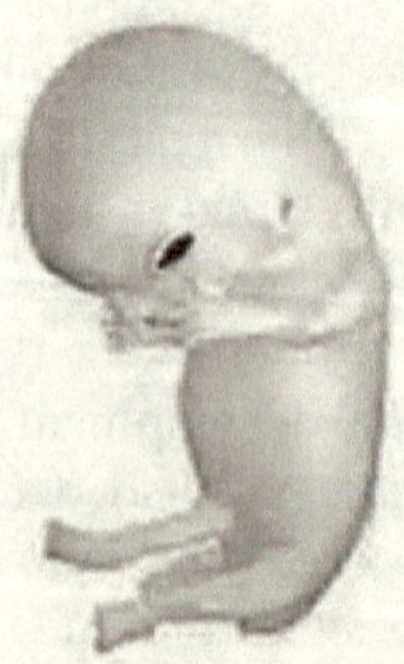

Fetus at 8 weeks after fertilization (gestational age of 10 weeks)

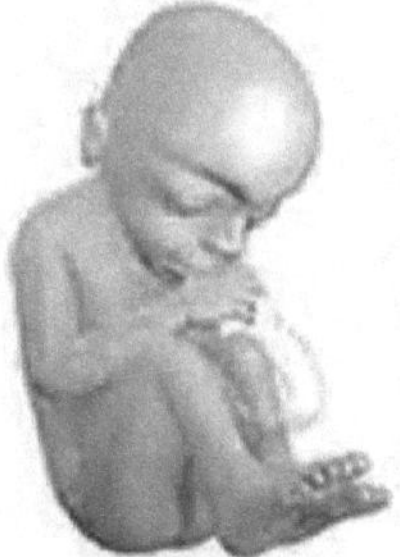

Fetus at 18 weeks after fertilization (gestational age of 20 weeks)

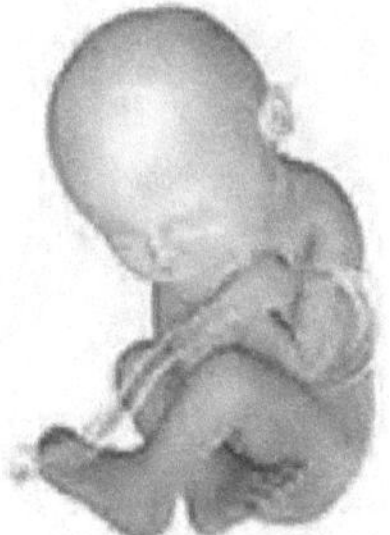

Fetus at 38 weeks after fertilization (gestational age of 40 weeks)

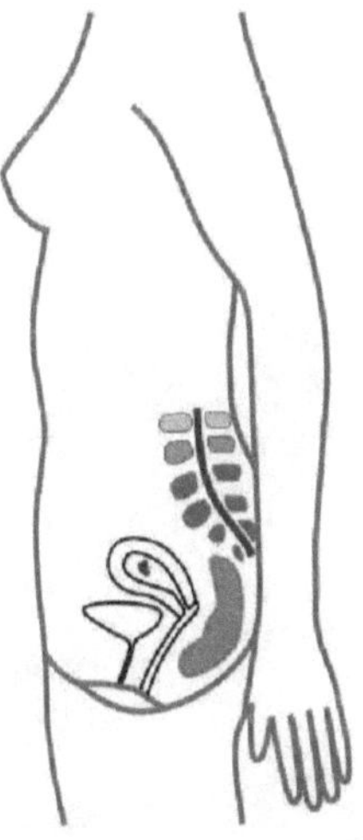

Relative size in 1st month (simplified illustration)

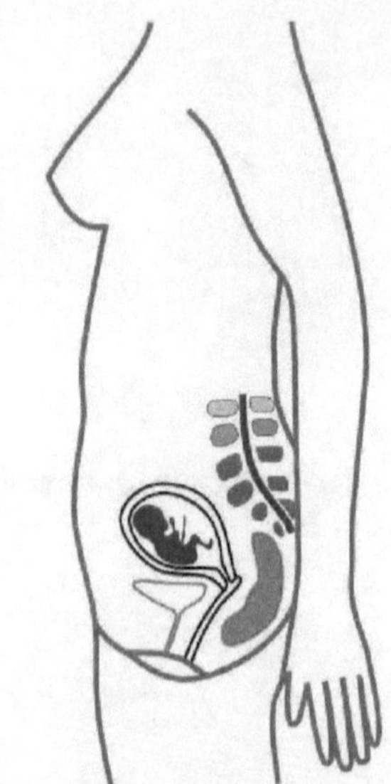

Relative size in 3rd month (simplified illustration)

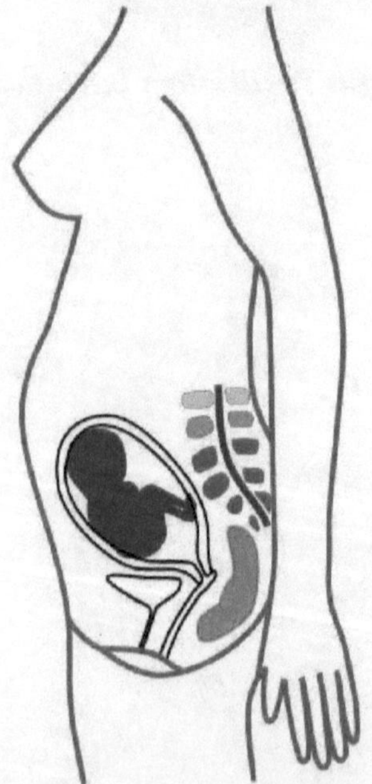

Relative size in 5th month (simplified illustration)

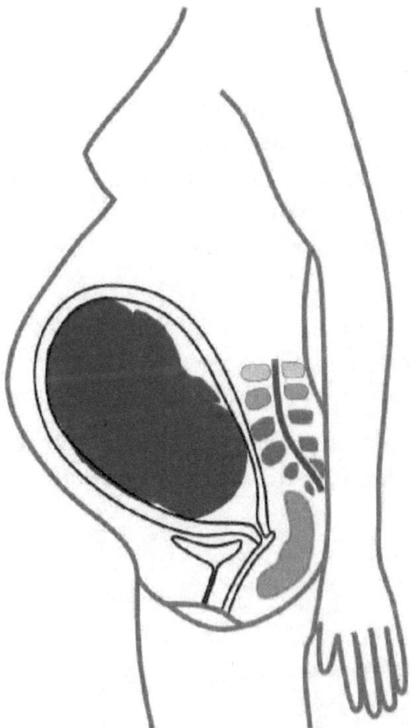

Relative size in 9th month (simplified illustration)

Maternal changes

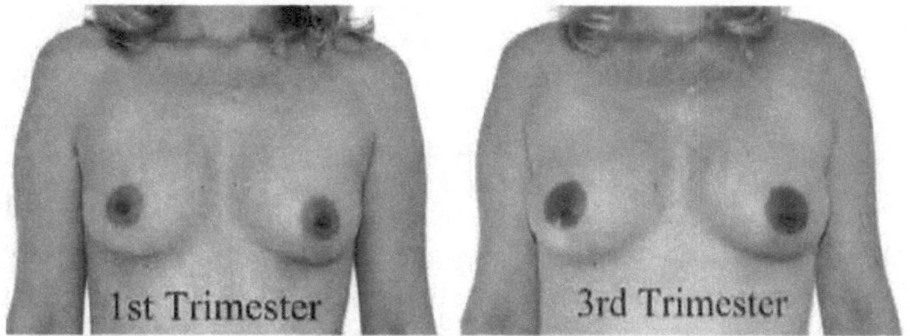

Breast changes as seen during pregnancy. The areolae are larger and darker.

During pregnancy, a woman undergoes many physiological changes, which are entirely normal, including behavioral, cardiovascular, hematologic, metabolic, renal, and respiratory changes. Increases in blood sugar, breathing, and cardiac output are all required.

Levels of progesterone and estrogens rise continually throughout pregnancy, suppressing the hypothalamic axis and therefore also the menstrual cycle. A full-term pregnancy at an early age reduces the risk of breast, ovarian and endometrial cancer and the risk declines further with each additional full-term pregnancy.

The fetus is genetically different from its mother, and can be viewed as an unusually successful allograft. The main reason for this success is increased immune tolerance during pregnancy.

Immune tolerance is the concept that the body is able to not mount an immune system response against certain triggers.

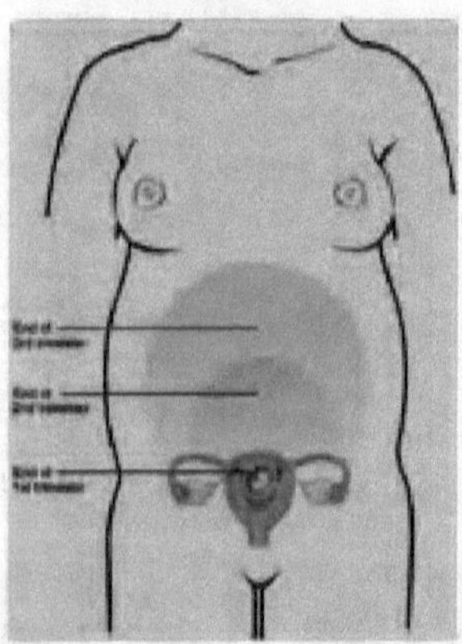

The uterus as it changes in size over the duration of the trimesters

During the first trimester, minute ventilation increases by 40%. The womb will grow to the size of a lemon by eight weeks. Many symptoms and discomforts of pregnancy like nausea and tender breasts appear in the first trimester.

During the second trimester, most women feel more energized, and begin to put on weight as the symptoms of morning sickness subside and eventually fade away. The uterus, the muscular organ that holds the developing fetus, can expand up to 20 times its normal size during pregnancy.

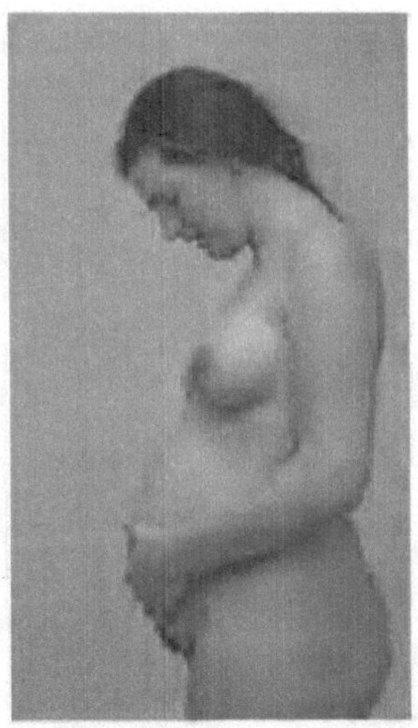

By the end of the second trimester, the expanding uterus has created a visible "baby bump". Although the breasts have been developing internally since the beginning of the pregnancy, most of the visible changes appear after this point.

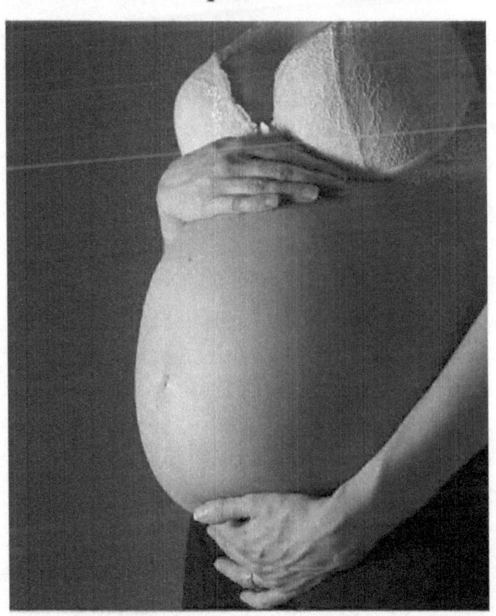

Pregnant woman in third trimester of pregnancy (last month)

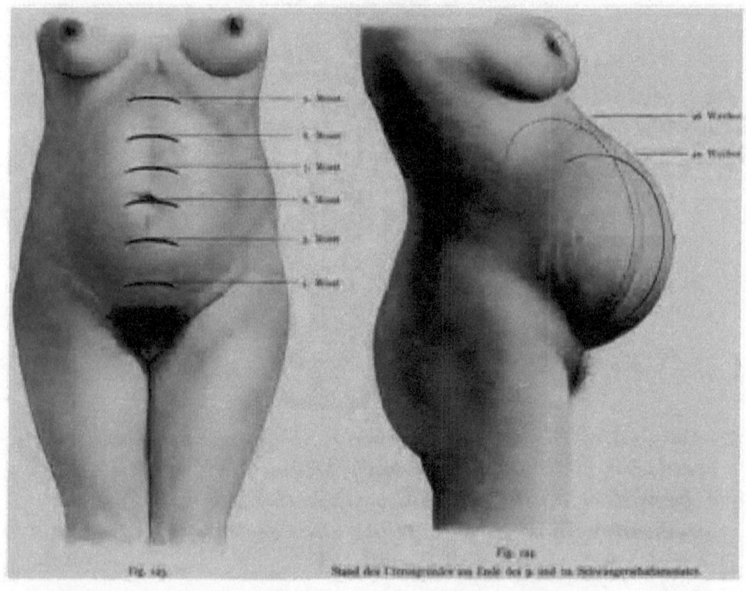

The uterus expands making up a larger and larger portion of the woman's abdomen. At left anterior view with months labeled, at right lateral view labeling the last 4 weeks. During the final stages of gestation before childbirth the fetus and uterus will drop to a lower position.

Braxton Hicks contractions are sporadic uterine contractions that may start around six weeks into a pregnancy however, they are usually not felt until the second or third trimester.

Final weight gain takes place during the third trimester, which is the most weight gain throughout the pregnancy. The woman's abdomen will transform in shape as it drops due to the fetus turning in a downward position ready for birth. During the second trimester, the woman's abdomen would have been upright, whereas in the third trimester it will drop down low.

The fetus moves regularly, and is felt by the woman. Fetal movement can become strong and be disruptive to the woman. The woman's navel will sometimes become convex, "popping" out, due to the expanding abdomen. Head engagement, also called "lightening" or "dropping" occurs as the fetal head descends into a cephalic presentation. While it relieves pressure on the upper abdomen and gives a renewed ease in breathing, it also severely reduces bladder capacity resulting in a need to void more frequently, and increases pressure on the pelvic floor and the rectum. It is not possible to predict when lightening occurs. In a first pregnancy it may happen a few weeks before the due date, though it may happen later or even not until labor begins, as is typical with subsequent pregnancies.

It is also during the third trimester that maternal activity and sleep positions may affect fetal development due to restricted blood flow. For instance, the enlarged uterus may impede blood flow by compressing the vena cava when lying flat, which is relieved by lying on the left side.

Childbirth

Childbirth, referred to as labor and delivery in the medical field, is the process whereby an infant is born.

A woman is considered to be in labour when she begins experiencing regular uterine contractions, accompanied by changes of her cervix—primarily effacement and dilation. While childbirth is widely experienced as painful, some women do report painless labours, while others find that concentrating on the birth helps to quicken labour and lessen the sensations. Most births are successful vaginal births, but sometimes complications arise and a woman may undergo a cesarean section.

During the time immediately after birth, both the mother and the baby are hormonally cued to bond, the mother through the release of oxytocin, a hormone also released during breastfeeding. Studies show that skin-to-skin contact between a mother and her newborn immediately after birth is beneficial for both the mother and baby.

A review done by the World Health Organization found that skin-to-skin contact between mothers and babies after birth reduces crying, improves mother–infant interaction, and helps mothers to breastfeed successfully. They recommend that neonates be allowed to bond with the mother during their first two hours after birth, the period that they tend to be more alert than in the following hours of early life.

Childbirth maturity stages

Stages of pregnancy term

Stage	Starts	Ends
Preterm	-	at 37 weeks
Early term	37 weeks	39 weeks
Full term	39 weeks	41 weeks
Late term	41 weeks	42 weeks
Postterm	42 weeks	-

In the ideal childbirth labor begins on its own when a woman is "at term". Events before completion of 37 weeks are considered preterm. Preterm birth is associated with a range of complications and should be avoided if possible.

Sometimes if a woman's water breaks or she has contractions before 39 weeks, birth is unavoidable. However, spontaneous birth after 37 weeks is considered term and is not associated with the same risks of a preterm birth.

Planned birth before 39 weeks by caesarean section or labor induction, although "at term", results in an increased risk of complications. This is from factors including underdeveloped lungs of newborns, infection due to underdeveloped immune system, feeding problems due to underdeveloped brain, and jaundice from underdeveloped liver.

Babies born between 39 and 41 weeks' gestation have better outcomes than babies born either before or after this range. This special time period is called "full term". Whenever possible, waiting for labor to begin on its own in this time period is best for the health of the mother and baby. The decision to perform an induction must be made after weighing the risks and benefits, but is safer after 39 weeks.

Events after 42 weeks are considered postterm. When a pregnancy exceeds 42 weeks, the risk of complications for both the woman and the fetus increases significantly. Therefore, in an otherwise uncomplicated pregnancy, obstetricians usually prefer to induce labour at some stage between 41 and 42 weeks.

Postnatal period

The postnatal period, also referred to as the *puerperium*, begins immediately after delivery and extends for about six weeks. During this period, the mother's body begins the return to pre-pregnancy conditions that includes changes in hormone levels and uterus size.

CARDIOVASCULAR AND LYMPHATIC SYSTEMS

During pregnancy the increasing needs of the growing fetus and of her own tissues throw an added burden on the mother's heart. The work that the heart does is measured by the amount of blood it expels per minute (the cardiac output). Rapid increase in the cardiac output occurs between the 9th and the 14th week of gestation.

During the period from the 28th to the 30th week, when the load is heaviest, the heart of a pregnant woman is doing 25 to 30 percent more work than it was doing before pregnancy.

As the time of delivery approaches, the heart's workload diminishes to some extent; when the baby is born, the load is approximately equal to what it was when the mother was in the nonpregnant state.

This decrease in cardiac output and cardiac work, which occurs in spite of the continued needs of the fetus and of the maternal tissues for blood-borne oxygen and nutriments, is explained by the more efficient way that the tissues draw on the mother's blood for oxygen and nourishment during the terminal weeks of pregnancy.

The position of the heart is changed to a greater or lesser degree during pregnancy. As the uterus enlarges, it elevates the diaphragm. This in turn pushes the heart upward, to the left, and somewhat forward, so that it is nearer the chest wall beneath the breast.

Near the end of gestation the large uterus may raise the heart until the latter lies almost at a right angle to the long axis of the woman's body. These changes, which also bring some rotation of the heart, vary considerably in different individuals. When present to a marked degree, they may give an examining physician the erroneous impression that a normal heart is considerably enlarged. Actually, in spite of its greater workload, a healthy heart enlarges little or not at all even during the midportion of pregnancy, when the load is greatest.

Changes in the position of the heart, the greater workload, the increased volume of blood that the heart expels per beat, the decreased viscosity of the blood, and the larger amount of blood in the woman's blood vessels will, in many women, cause some distortion of the sounds that the physician hears when listening to a patient's heart with a stethoscope.

Such distorted sounds, called "functional" murmurs (as distinguished from "organic" murmurs, which may be present when the heart is diseased), do not indicate that anything is amiss, although they may be sufficiently atypical to cause the obstetrician to refer the patient to a cardiologist for evaluation. Pregnancy sometimes produces minor changes in the electrocardiogram, but these changes are within normal limits.

Such is the ability of the heart to respond to an increased workload that even the pregnant woman with serious heart disease, given proper care and without an unexpected complication, will usually go through her pregnancy and delivery without a catastrophe. She may, however, encounter difficulty when she tries to cope with the stress of caring for her family after the baby is born.

Normal pregnancy does not increase the mother's blood pressure. Indeed, a slight lowering of the blood pressure is commonly noted during the course of the pregnancy. Any notable rise in a pregnant woman's blood pressure is reason for alertness on the part of her physician, and, if it continues to rise, for concern; it usually foretells the onset of preeclampsia.

The pulse rate is a trifle more rapid during pregnancy, reflecting the more rapid heartbeat that is necessary in order to move the larger volume of blood present. The rate at which blood flows through the myriad of small blood vessels in the skin (the peripheral circulation) is accelerated during pregnancy, leading to the elevated skin temperature, the tendency to perspire, and, in part, to the redness of the palms and the tiny dilated blood vessels in some women as their pregnancies progress.

The most notable change in the circulatory system during pregnancy, other than those described in the heart, is a slowing of the blood flow in the lower extremities.

With this decrease in the rate of flow there is an increase in the pressure within the veins and some stasis—stagnation—of the blood in the legs. These changes, which are believed to be caused primarily by the pressure of the uterus on the large blood vessels in the pelvis, are progressive during pregnancy and disappear after delivery.

They also are thought to be caused in part by the marked increase in the amounts of the hormones estrogen and progesterone in the circulating blood. Increased venous pressure, slowing of the rate of venous flow, and partial stasis of the blood in the veins are major factors in causing the swelling of the legs and the varicose (abnormally dilated) veins of the lower legs that are commonly present near the end of pregnancy.

The lymphatic vessels of the pregnant woman's pelvis become enlarged in response to the increased amount of tissue fluid in the engorged pelvic organs. As the uterus grows in size, it presses on these channels, causing impairment of the lymphatic drainage from the woman's legs, with resultant swelling and distention of her feet and legs.

Although some fluid almost invariably collects in the feet, ankles, and legs near the time of delivery, sudden swelling of the feet and legs or a notable increase in swelling may be an early signal of impending preeclampsia, a serious disorder of pregnancy that is discussed below. Generalized swelling—i.e., swelling of the hands, face, and other parts of the body—is a cause for serious concern.

RESPIRATORY TRACT

One would expect that, as the uterus grows larger and pushes the diaphragm up, it would interfere with breathing, but the lungs actually work as efficiently as they do in the nonpregnant state. This is due to a change in the shape of the chest cavity during pregnancy; the chest diameter increases as its height decreases, so that there is actually a slight increase in the space that the lungs occupy.

The amount of air drawn in and expelled per minute by the lungs increases progressively during pregnancy. Immediately before delivery the number of breaths per minute is approximately twice what it is after the baby is born. This, like so many of the other changes in the mother's body, is an adaptation of one of her vital functions that is necessary to supply her tissues and those of the growing fetus with increasing amounts of oxygen.

GASTROINTESTINAL TRACT

A number of alterations, often causing more or less distress, occur in the physical condition and functions of the gastrointestinal tract during pregnancy.

Disturbances of the sensations of taste and smell, relatively common during early months of gestation, are often accompanied by a dislike of odours and a distaste of foods formerly found to be agreeable. The inflammation of the mouth and gums that some pregnant women complain of is more often caused by poor oral hygiene, by vitamin deficiencies, or by anemia than by the pregnancy itself.

Hydrochloric acid and pepsin, adequate amounts of which are necessary for satisfactory digestion, are produced by the stomach in decreased amounts during pregnancy.

This decrease in the amount of acid in the stomach may explain some of the otherwise inexplicable anemias that occasionally occur during the course of an otherwise seemingly normal pregnancy. During pregnancy the stomach muscles lose some of their tone and become more flabby, and the contractility of the stomach is reduced.

As a result, the time it takes for the stomach to empty its contents into the intestinal tract is prolonged. As pregnancy progresses, the stomach is pushed upward; near term it lies like a flabby pouch across the top of the uterus instead of hanging downward, as it normally does, in a semivertical position. The loss of tone of the stomach muscles, the decrease in stomach acidity, and the change in position of the stomach are conducive to the flow of intestinal contents back into the stomach.

These disturbances in gastric function are responsible, in part at least, for the intolerance for fatty foods, the indigestion, the discomfort felt in the upper part of the abdomen, and the heartburn experienced by most pregnant women at some time during their pregnancies.

The musculature not only of the stomach but also of the entire intestinal tract loses much of its tonicity. As a result, peristalsis, the series of wavelike movements of the intestines, is slowed, the length of time it takes food to pass through the intestinal tract is prolonged, and there is more or less stagnation of the intestinal contents.

Constipation and hemorrhoids that cause rectal pain and bleeding are common complaints during pregnancy. The constipation is caused by lack of tone of the intestinal tract and stagnation of the bowel contents.

Pregnant women may also lose the urge to defecate because of the pressure of the uterus on the lower bowel and inhibition of a reflex stimulus, known as the gastrocolic reflex, from the stomach to the rectum.

The latter mechanism, which depends on normal stomach function, is responsible for the increased activity of the lower bowel that follows increased stomach activity, such as that induced by eating. It is this reflex that causes many persons to feel a desire to defecate within an hour or so after eating a full meal. Hemorrhoids—greatly enlarged or varicose veins in the lower rectum—that appear during pregnancy are due to constipation, to stasis of blood in the pelvic veins, and to pressure by the enlarging uterus on the blood vessels in the pelvis.

Liver

The liver, which plays an essential role in many of the vital processes—processes as diverse as participating in the metabolism of nutriments and vitamins and the elimination of the waste products of metabolism—changes anatomically and functionally during pregnancy to meet the added load placed on it by the maternal organism, the enlarging uterus, and, to a lesser extent, the growing fetus.

The liver's ability to synthesize proteins and to supply minerals and nutriments is augmented in response to the increased requirements of the mother's tissue and the fetus. The liver adjusts to the greatly augmented amounts of hormones circulating in the mother's blood during pregnancy.

It helps to dispose of or detoxify the larger amounts of waste material produced by the metabolic processes in the growing fetus, the enlarging uterus, and the mother's tissues. Furthermore, the blood vessels in the liver enlarge to accommodate the larger amount of blood in the mother's blood vessels.

At the same time, the liver must compensate for the larger number of circulating red blood cells. In response to these demands, the liver increases in size and weight, and its blood vessels become larger, but otherwise its anatomic structure changes relatively little during pregnancy.

The hormones produced by the placenta and the metabolic changes in the maternal organism, rather than the fetus, are the factors responsible not only for the increased work the liver does but also for many of the physical and functional alterations that appear during gestation.

URINARY TRACT

Changes that take place in the bladder and the urethra during pregnancy are attributable to relaxation of the muscles supporting these structures, to change in position, and to pressure.

The uterus lies over the bladder and presses upon it during early pregnancy. Later the uterus rises out of the pelvis. As the uterus grows larger and moves upward, the bladder is pushed forward and pulled upward.

The urethra, the tube through which urine is discharged from the bladder, is stretched and distorted. As these distortions take place, the wall of the bladder becomes thickened, the blood vessels become enlarged, and fluid collects in the tissues forming the wall of the bladder. The results are swelling, stasis of blood in the blood vessels, and some mechanical inflammation of the bladder wall.

The woman is likely to urinate frequently during the early months of pregnancy when the heavy uterus presses on the bladder. Frequent urination is less common during midpregnancy, but it recurs after the baby descends into the pelvis near the time of delivery.

As the bladder and urethra are pulled upward and distorted by the growing uterus, the stretched muscles that control urination are less efficient, and the woman may lose some urine involuntarily when she coughs, sneezes, or laughs; this is known as stress incontinence.

The swelling, mechanical inflammation, and stasis of blood in the blood vessels of the bladder near the end of pregnancy are conducive to bladder infection, a symptom of which is pain on urination.

A microscopic examination of the urine is necessary to differentiate between the effect of pregnancy on bladder function and the symptoms caused by a bladder infection. An untreated bladder infection may lead to serious urinary tract troubles later.

Changes in the structure and function of the ureters, the two rubbery, spaghetti-like tubes that carry urine from the kidneys to the bladder, are present in 80 percent of all pregnancies.

As pregnancy progresses, each ureter becomes larger, so that it lies in multiple broad curves rather than forming an almost straight line downward from the kidney. In addition, both ureters, but particularly the right one, become greatly dilated, so that the urine flows very slowly or collects in them.

The funnellike part of the kidney, called the kidney pelvis, also becomes dilated. With this dilation of the kidney pelvis and the ureters there is also a loss of tonicity or contractility in the pelvis of the kidney and the ureters.

This loss of tonicity during pregnancy is similar to that mentioned in the description of the changes in the intestinal tract. Since it is the contractility of peristalsis within the ureter that propels urine downward from the kidney into the bladder, stasis of urine in the ureter is accentuated during the pregnancy.

In the nonpregnant state the hydrostatic pressure in the kidney is greater than that in the bladder; during pregnancy the situation is reversed. This change of pressure further increases the stasis of urine in the ureter and kidney pelvis. As a result, bladder infections are more serious during pregnancy, because they are more likely to involve the kidney. After delivery the ureters rapidly return to their normal condition.

The kidney of a healthy person selectively filters and secretes water, sodium, potassium, chlorides, protein, and other substances from the blood. It then reabsorbs water and essential elements in amounts that are needed to maintain the fluid, electrolytic, and other chemical balances in the body.

It also filters waste products of metabolism from the blood and excretes them in the urine. During pregnancy the kidney continues to carry on these functions. The workload placed on it, however, is greater because of the increase in the amount of water and blood and in the rate of metabolism during gestation.

In early pregnancy, secretion of large amounts of dilute urine of decreased acidity, together with pressure of the uterus on the bladder, causes frequency of urination and nocturnal voiding. Less urine is excreted toward the end of pregnancy. The storage of large amounts of nitrogen, as part of the metabolism of proteins, causes a decrease in the urinary excretion of urea and of total nitrogen during gestation.

Although many healthy pregnant women occasionally show a trace of protein (albumin) in their urine, the detection of even small amounts of protein in the urine is a cause for alertness on the part of a physician, because anything more than an extremely small amount may be the first signal of impending preeclampsia or kidney disease, both of which are serious complications.

The kidney's ability to reabsorb sugar (glucose) is lower during pregnancy, and for this reason many pregnant women have transient periods during which their urine contains small amounts of glucose; such women have unimpaired ability to metabolize carbohydrates and have normal sugar levels in the blood.

Glucose in the urine also may be the first sign that a person has diabetes mellitus, however; consequently, a pregnant woman whose urine contains traces of glucose is tested to make sure that she can metabolize sugar normally.

The preceding discussion of kidney function illustrates the need for a pregnant woman to be under a health-care provider's care, an essential part of which is periodic examination of her urine for protein, sugar, pus, bacteria, and other abnormal constituents.

BLOOD

The total amount of blood in a pregnant woman's body has increased by approximately 25 percent by the time of delivery. The increase is accounted for by the augmented volume of blood plasma (the liquid part of the blood), which is caused by fluid retention, plus an increase in the total number of red blood cells.

Additional blood is needed to fill the large vessels of the uterus. Also, more blood is required to carry the oxygen and nutriments needed by the fetus and the maternal tissues and to carry away waste products. Furthermore, it is a protective reserve in case of hemorrhage during delivery.

During pregnancy the blood-forming organs, such as the bone marrow, make more erythrocytes, or red blood cells, which carry iron and oxygen.

Despite this, there is usually a decrease in a pregnant woman's blood cell count—the number of red cells per cubic millimetre of blood—because the amount of blood plasma increases approximately 30 percent, while the total number of red blood cells increases by only about 20 percent. This results in apparent anemia.

With these changes, the viscosity of the blood decreases and the hematocrit, which measures the relative amounts of liquid and solid constituents in the blood, is lower. Usually there is a moderate increase in the number of white blood cells per cubic millimetre during early pregnancy; this increase disappears during the latter part of pregnancy. If a pregnant woman is otherwise healthy and receives adequate available iron for the production of hemoglobin, her red blood cell count does not ordinarily fall below 3,750,000 cells per cubic millimetre, her hemoglobin below 13.5 grams per 100 cubic millimetres of blood, and her hematocrit below 35. (Normal values for nonpregnant women are 4,200,000–5,400,000 cells, 13.8–14.2 grams hemoglobin, and 37–47 hematocrit.) Physicians usually make blood counts for their pregnant patients every two months because of the need for repeated evaluation.

Endocrine system

Most of the endocrine glands become larger, and some display alterations in function, during pregnancy; they all revert to a normal state after delivery.

The anterior lobe of the pituitary gland increases in size during pregnancy, but the production of pituitary gonadotropins, the gonad-stimulating hormones, ceases soon after the placenta begins to produce chorionic gonadotropins. The pituitary continues to secrete the hormones that stimulate the other endocrine glands. Near term, as the mother's estrogen level drops, a milk-stimulating hormone, prolactin, is produced by the pituitary. The posterior lobe of the pituitary gland does not change in size or weight during pregnancy.

The thyroid gland enlarges moderately, but there is no true increase in thyroid function during gestation. The parathyroid glands also increase in size during pregnancy but presumably are not otherwise affected by it.

The part of the pancreas that secretes insulin, the islets of Langerhans, becomes larger. Whatever increase in function is displayed may be assumed to be a balanced response to the body's demand for the products of carbohydrate metabolism. The level of plasma insulin or of insulin-like substances in the plasma is higher during pregnancy, and the destruction of insulin is also more rapid.

The blood and urinary levels of 17-hydroxycorticosteroids, hormones that affect protein, fat, and carbohydrate metabolism and that are produced by the adrenal glands, rise during pregnancy; but there is no increased effect from the hormones, because their higher level is more than offset by the increased levels of transcortin, a protein that inactivates them. As gestation progresses, there is an elevation in the secretion of aldosterone, an adrenal hormone that plays a role in the retention of salt and water in the body. It has been suggested that this is a protective mechanism to counterbalance the tendency for progesterone to cause the excretion of sodium ions in the urine.

Skin

Pregnancy usually causes an increase in the secretion of the oil and sweat glands in the skin. Body odours may become more pronounced. Many women notice that their hair becomes thinner and drier and their nails more brittle.

Others may develop an increased amount of facial and body hair. The "mask of pregnancy" seen particularly in brunettes is a deposit of brownish pigment in the skin of the forehead, the cheeks, and the nose. Puffiness and thickening of her skin may cause the pregnant woman's face to appear coarse and almost masculine. Increased pigmentation, particularly of the smooth skin about the nipples (the areolas of the breasts) and the vulva, is almost universal.

Bright red discoloration of the palms of the hands and tiny spiderweb-like red blood vessels in the skin of the arms or face are not unusual during pregnancy. Many of these changes are thought to be associated with the greatly increased levels of estrogen in the mother's bloodstream. Most of the changes disappear after delivery.

"Stretch marks," which appear on the breasts and abdomen during pregnancy, are due to the tearing of the elastic tissues in the skin that accompanies enlargement of the breasts, distention of the abdomen, and the deposition of subcutaneous fat. They are pink or purplish red lines during pregnancy.

The lines become permanent scarlike marks after delivery. Some women never develop stretch marks despite bearing several children; others lose most of the tone in their skin after one pregnancy.

Stretch marks cannot be considered evidence that a woman has borne a child, however, because they sometimes are seen in women who have not been pregnant.

METABOLIC CHANGES

Metabolic changes during pregnancy are among the many adjustments that the mother's organs make to meet the requirements created by the increase in her own breast and genital tissues and the growth of the conceptus (the fetus and afterbirth). In addition, reserves must be established to meet the demands that will be put on her body during pregnancy, delivery, and the postdelivery period.

The basal metabolic rate

The amount of oxygen consumed is an index of the pregnant woman's metabolism when she is at rest—her basal metabolism. The rate begins to rise during the third month of pregnancy and may double the normal rate (+10 percent) by the time of delivery.

The rate rises in specific proportion to the size of the fetus and represents the effects of the mother's activities plus those of the fetus and the uterine structures. An elevation of the basal metabolic rate (BMR) to 20 or 25 percent during pregnancy is not an indication of an overly active thyroid gland.

Weight

The early part of pregnancy usually is accompanied by moderate weight loss caused by the woman's lack of appetite and in some cases nausea and vomiting. Between the third and the ninth month of pregnancy most women gain about 9 kilograms (20 pounds) or more.

Ideally, during pregnancy, body weight is gained at the rate of about 0.5 kilogram (1 pound) per week for a total of not more than 9 to 11.5 kilograms (20 to 25 pounds). In an average pregnancy the infant, the afterbirth, and the fluid in the uterus weigh about 4.5 kilograms (10 pounds).

The uterus and the breasts together weigh approximately 2.25 kilograms (5 pounds). The remaining 2.25 kilograms consist of stored fluids and fat. Weight gain exceeding 11.5 kilograms usually represents fat and fluids that are in excess of the reserve requirements for a normal pregnancy. A woman loses approximately 7 kilograms (15 pounds) at delivery, and another 2.25 kilograms of stored fluid are eliminated as the uterus shrinks.

She does not lose many additional kilograms during the weeks following the delivery of the baby unless she limits her caloric intake. Fat stored during pregnancy is lost more slowly than stored fluids, proteins, and carbohydrates.

Excessive weight gain during pregnancy is a matter of concern for both the patient and the doctor. Although it may be only the result of overeating, it may be caused by a disturbance in metabolism and by an abnormal retention of fluids and salts.

In the latter instance it may be the first sign of preeclampsia. An increase of 20 or more pounds above recommended weight gain based on prepregnancy body mass index is associated with a significant increase in the risk of complications at the time of delivery, including eclampsia, maternal heart failure, and maternal need for ventilation.

Protein

During pregnancy, nitrogen, derived from the metabolism of ingested protein, is needed for growth of the fetus, the placenta, the uterus, and the mother's breasts and other tissues. A considerable amount of nitrogen also is required for the increase in the mother's red cell volume and blood plasma.

The fetus's demand for nitrogen is slight at first, but during the last month of pregnancy it acquires almost half of its total protein. In the process of accumulating this store and of building a reserve for the period after delivery, the woman who is on an adequate diet retains between two and three grams of nitrogen daily during her pregnancy; by term she and the fetus will have acquired approximately 500 grams (about 1.1 pounds) of nitrogen.

Carbohydrates

During pregnancy greater quantities of blood are being processed through the kidneys, but the kidneys are incapable of reabsorbing increased amounts of sugar. Consequently, a lower level of sugar in the blood is tolerated, and slight amounts of sugar are excreted in the urine.

During pregnancy the level of sugar in the blood after fasting is slightly lower, probably because there is less usable insulin in the blood to regulate the sugar metabolism. Oral glucose-tolerance tests show a prolonged elevation of blood sugar after ingestion of glucose; this may be an indication that carbohydrate use is less rapid or that the absorption of glucose from the gastrointestinal tract is slower.

Glucose-tolerance tests that depend on injection of the sugar solution into the veins show no difference between nonpregnant and pregnant nondiabetic women. A few women demonstrate diabetes for the first time when they are pregnant, a condition referred to as gestational diabetes. This occurs because pregnancy taxes insulin productivity in women with a marginal pancreatic islet reserve, so that diabetes may first become evident during gestation.

Fat

The total blood lipids average 600 to 700 milligrams per hundred millilitres of blood in the nonpregnant woman. They increase to approximately 900 to 1,000 milligrams per hundred millilitres of blood during the latter part of pregnancy.

This increase, which involves all the lipid fractions, has not been explained, but it is worthy of notice that the gain in fat reaches its acme during the period that the fetus acquires most of its adipose (fatty) tissue.

Water

Pregnancy is characterized by increases in the amount of body water and in the total volume of body fluid. During pregnancy between 3,500 and 4,000 millilitres of fluid (about 3.2 to 3.6 quarts) will be added to that already present in the tissues of a healthy woman.

The uterus, the placenta, the amniotic fluid, and the fetus each account for approximately equal amounts. In addition to the water that increases blood volume, there is also added fluid in the mother's muscles, her pelvic soft tissues, her breasts, and her other tissues.

Toward the end of pregnancy a considerable amount of retained fluid accumulates in the woman's lower extremities. It is this fluid that produces the pitting and swelling of the legs that many normally pregnant women display during the month or two before delivery.

Retention of large amounts of electrolytes, particularly sodium, accompanies the increase in the amount of body fluids. Approximately 12 grams of sodium are retained monthly.

In addition to a positive sodium balance, there is a positive chloride and potassium balance during pregnancy.

As a result, additional water is required to maintain the balance of the solution of sodium, chloride, and potassium in the blood, in the fluid of the spaces between the tissue cells, and within the cells themselves.

Not all of the sodium, however, goes into fluid. Some of it is stored, and some replaces potassium in the cells.

A number of factors contribute to a positive sodium balance, which in turn leads to retention of fluid; these include alterations in the kidneys' excretion of sodium and water; increased retention of water in the pregnant woman's legs; the large amounts of hormones, particularly estrogen, that the placenta secretes; and the secretion of adrenal hormones, especially aldosterone. The latter, in particular, reduces the kidneys' secretion of sodium.

Because sodium and water interact with each other, whatever contributes to the retention of one leads to the retention of the other. Generalized swelling appears when the accumulation of sodium and water becomes too great.

Minerals

The pregnant woman's reserves and intake of iron and calcium must be enough not only for her own needs but also for those of the fetus. An increase in serum copper levels occurs during pregnancy. The mother has some phosphorus reserve but must acquire enough from her diet to supply her own tissues and those of the fetus. The use of phosphorus and that of calcium are interdependent, so that the use of phosphorus depends on the calcium intake.

Bibliography

Ausubel, D.P.: *Theory and problems of child development.* New York: Grune & Stratton, 1958.

Bloomfield, P.: *Moral Reality,* New York: Oxford University Press, 2001.

Bower, T. C. R.: *Development in infancy.* San Francisco: Freeman and Co., 1974.

Brown SS. *Prenatal Care: Reaching Mothers, Reaching Infants.* Washington, DC: National Academy Press, 1998.

Browne, J, and Dixon, G.: *Antenatal Care,* Churchill Livingstone, London, 1978.

Bulygin and Niniluoto, *Man, Law and Modern Forms of Life,* D. Reidel Publishing Company, Boston (1985)

Calder, A. and Dunlop, W.: *High Risk Pregnancy,* Butterworth Heinemann, Oxford, UK, 1992.

Canguilhem, G. *The Normal and the Pathological,* C.R.Fawcett, New York: Zone Books, 1991. .

Carel, H., *Illness: The Cry of the Flesh,* Dublin: Acumen, 2008. .

Carter, K. C., *The Rise of Causal Theories of Disease in Women,* Aldershot and Burlington, VT: Ashgate, 2003. .

Chalmers I, Enkin M, Keirse M. *Effective care in pregnancy and childbirth.* Oxford: Oxford University Press, 1989.

Coles, Robert. *The Moral Intelligence of Children: How to Raise a Moral Child.* New York: Random House, 1997.

Cook, Rachel, *Surrogate Motherhood: International Perspective,* Hart Publishing, New York (2003)

Culver, C. M. and Gert, B., *Philosophy in Medicine,* New York: Oxford University Press, 1982. .

Davey, D.: *Hypertensive disorders of pregnancy,* Churchill Livingstone, London, 1985.

El- Mesellawy, Y.: *Essential Obstetrics.* University Book Centre, Cairo, 1992.

Erminio, Peter Volpe, *Test-tube Conception: A Blend of Love and Science,* Mercer University Press, Georgia, USA (1987)

Field, Martha A., *Surrogate Motherhood: The Legal and Human Issues,* Harvard University Press, London (1990)

Friedman, E.: *Obstetrical Decision Making.* B.C.Decker Inc. New Jersey, USA, 1982.

Gadamer, H-G., *The Enigma of Women Health,* Stanford: Stanford University Press, 1996. .

Green, J. A., *Prescribing by Numbers,* Baltimore: Johns Hopkins, 2007. .

Hibbard, B.: *Principles of Obstetrics,* Butterworth International Ed., London, 1988.

Horwitz, A. V., *Creating Mental Illness in Women,* Chicago: University of Chicago Press, 2002. .

Kitcher, P., *The Lives To Come: The Genetic Revolution and Human Possibilities,* revised edition, New York: Simon & Schuster. 1997. .

Law, R.: *Ultrasound in Clinical Obstetrics.* John Wright & Sons Ltd., Bristol, UK, 1980.

Layne, Linda, *Transformative Motherhood: On Giving and Getting in a Consumer Culture,* New York University Press, New York (1999)

Nordenfelt, L., *On the Nature of Health: An Action-Theoretic Perspective,* 2nd edition, Dordrecht: Kluwer, 1995. .

Piaget, J.: *The Construction of Reality in the Child.* New York: Basic Books, 1954.

Rae, Scott B. *The Ethics of Commercial Surrogate Motherhood: Brave New Families?* Westport, CT: Praeger, 1994.

Reznek, L., *The Nature of Disease,* New York: Routledge, 1987. .

Stewart, K.: *The scond stage, In: Progress in Obstetrics and Gynaecology,* Churchill Livingstone, London, 1984.

Stirrat, G.: *Immunology of Pregnancy,* Churchill Livingstone, London, 1985.

Taylor, J.: *Science and the Supernatural. An investigation of paranormal phenomena.* London: Granada, 1980.

Thagard. P., *How Scientists Explain in Women Disease,* Princeton: Princeton University Press. 1999. .

Waters, Brent. *Reproductive Technology: Towards a Theology of Procreative Stewardship.* Cleveland: Pilgrim Press, 2001.

Index

❑❑❑